RUNNING, EATING, THINKING

RUNNING, EATING, THINKING

A Vegan Anthology

MARTIN ROWE, EDITOR

LANTERN BOOKS / NEW YORK

A Division of Booklight Inc.

2014
Lantern Books
128 Second Place
Brooklyn, NY 11231
www.lanternbooks.com

Printed in the United States of America

ISBN: (pbk) 978-1-59056-348-9, (ebook) 978-1-59056-425-7

Library of Congress Cataloguing-in-Publication information is available.

Contents

Foreword

Paul Shapiro

"You may not run again—but we're gonna do everything we can to make sure that doesn't happen."

I absorbed the doctor's words, looking up at an x-ray of my left kneecap, or rather my left kneecaps—plural. About two-thirds sat on top of my quad; the other third just above my shin. Gazing at the gulf between the two bone fragments, I joked to the doctor it was like Moses had parted the "Red Knee." Stupid one, but he chuckled, probably out of sympathy.

The spot in which my kneecap normally parked itself of course had felt bone-hard for the prior three decades. Now, its consistency more closely resembled a pack of energy gel that long-distance runners use to fuel themselves—something I knew nothing about at the time.

Just an hour earlier I'd imagined that my kneecap was "merely" dislocated—not broken—and that it would need to be slid back into place. Images of Mel Gibson in *Lethal Weapon* popping his shoulder in and out of its socket flashed in my mind, and after tempting fate by trying to even lightly manipulate the injury, I resolved that I wasn't likely to make this the same kind of DIY procedure Officer Riggs did.

And now, there it was: plain as day on the brightly backlit x-ray in front of me. My mother had always warned me that playing football was dangerous, and I usually took her counsel of caution to be that of the stereotypical Jewish mother: worried and overprotective, but with good intention. She almost didn't believe the news when I called her before the surgery, thinking perhaps it was a prank. It was only when I texted her a photo of the x-ray that she began the panic. "Breaking kneecaps is what the mob does; what kind of collision did you get yourself into?!"

"Mom, I'm not panicking; why are you?"

Logic is often no consolation to a worried mother learning about her child's catastrophic injury.

Twelve months and three surgeries later, along with innumerable torturous—in the most literal sense of the word—physical therapy sessions, I thought perhaps it was time to test this whole running thing out. I'd never run more than a few miles, and certainly didn't consider myself a "runner." But the thought of being told that it was possible I may never be able to do something had its effect—and so my journey began.

Being vegan since 1993, I'd certainly read much literature about the amazing healing properties of various whole plants, and I started consuming potent anti-inflammatory foods (like cayenne and turmeric) in order to prevent my knee from sending very unwelcome pain signals to my brain. At first, I could run for about a minute without debilitating pain. Then a few minutes. Eventually, I started running 5 and 10K races. My times may not have been impressive, but the fact that I could run at all seemed to me somewhat as if Moses may have worked another minor miracle.

It was reading Rich Roll's *Finding Ultra* that persuaded me that perhaps my body was capable of a lot more than I expected, and that the power of health-promoting vegan foods to repair us shouldn't be underestimated. That realization led me on a journey that has culminated in my running the Marine Corps Marathon as well as numerous half-marathons, all through which my kneecap has happily remained functional. (For those wondering, not only did I let my surgeon know, I mailed him my marathon bib, which he now proudly hangs in his office for other patients to see.)

The experience certainly reinforced for me that we're capable of much greater achievements than most of us ever allow ourselves to envision. That seems true to me athletically; but, far more importantly, it seems true for our movement's efforts to improve our world.

My career is waging campaigns to help farm animals, and often the type of battles we're facing seem much tougher than the final quarter-mile of the Marine Corps Marathon—notoriously and cruelly uphill. The animal protection movement is tiny compared to our multi-billion dollar adversaries in the animal agribusiness industry, yet I know that we can not only challenge them, but we can beat them. I know it because we do it time and time again.

When our movement has gone up against the factory farmers in ballot measures—in states like Florida, Arizona, and California—despite multi-million-dollar campaigns against us, we've decisively won every time. During our 2008 Proposition 2 campaign in California—to ban gestation crates, battery cages, and veal crates—political pundits laughed us off when we announced we'd be taking on the ag industry in the nation's largest ag state. Yet in the end, two-thirds of voters sided with animals, not their abusers; we won by a landslide.

Similarly, the entire concept of vegan eating, once foreign and on the social margins, is now firmly cemented into the mainstream, with cultural icons from Ellen DeGeneres and Oprah Winfrey to Bill Clinton and Bill Gates extolling the benefits of eating more plants and fewer animals. When I became a vegan more than twenty years ago, people didn't know what the word meant, let alone how to pronounce it. Now, little could be further from the truth, and per capita animal consumption in the U.S. is declining for the first time, and consequently, so is the number of animals who we're raising and killing for food.

All marathons begin with a single step, and our movement has a long way to go. But we've taken impressively important strides in recent years—progress that many would have considered nearly impossible in the very recent past. I firmly believe down to my bones (including my left kneecap) that we will create a new, much more humane society, in which our relationship with other animals will no longer be based solely on violence and domination, but rather upon compassion and respect.

I know that type of a world may seem impossible. It may seem just too farfetched considering where we are now. But lots of incredible outcomes have at one point seemed impossible.

A historian once told Gandhi that his dream of freeing India from British rule was impossible. The Mahatma famously replied, "Sir, your job is to teach history. Ours is to make it."

And that's our task in the animal protection movement: to make history.

Coming back from a broken kneecap to run marathons may not be historic in any way. But the improbability of such an outcome serves as a helpful metaphor for the seemingly improbable task our movement is trying to accomplish. Surely we have massive hurdles to overcome, but slowly and steadily we're running past them, and will only continue to get faster.

PAUL SHAPIRO *is the vice president of farm animal protection at The Humane Society of the United States. You can follow him at http://twitter. com/pshapiro.*

Introduction

Martin Rowe

In 1992, I was in graduate school, undergoing the initiatory rites appropriate for attaining a master's degree in religious studies, when Indiana University Press published an anthology with the intriguing title of *Cooking, Eating, Thinking: Transformative Philosophies of Food*. My graduate thesis aimed to analyze animals and food in the Bible, which one wag noted could be summarized as one long argument about the purity or otherwise of what goes into or comes out of one's mouth. So Deane Curtin and Lisa Heldke's volume seemed just what I needed to stimulate my tastebuds.

Cooking, Eating, Thinking's opening paragraph begins as follows:

> Normally an anthology comes "after the fact"; it provides a retrospective view of territory that has already been mapped. This anthology departs from that convention. It attempts to establish the existence of a philosophical subject matter and to provide various ways of approaching that subject matter. . . . We intend for this work to stand as a multi-voiced argument for the existence of a domain of philosophic inquiry; it is a *reader* in the philosophy of food. (CET xiii)

As we'll see, *Running, Eating, Thinking: A Vegan Anthology* owes many ideas to *Cooking, Eating, Thinking*. But more than anything else, the anthology you're reading—like its forebear—aims to "establish the existence of a philosophical subject matter." It recognizes its own incompleteness and invites further and deeper exploration of what, on the face of it, may seem only tangentially related activities.

In his introduction to *Cooking, Eating, Thinking*, Deane Curtin acknowledges that one reason for philosophers' relative silence about eating, at least within the Western tradition, is that food in particular and the desires and needs of the body in general have been considered not only inappropriate subjects for but positively antithetical to the business of thinking. Curtin quotes Socrates' question in Plato's *Phaedo*: "Do you think that it is right for a philosopher to concern himself with the so-called pleasures connected with food and drink?"

> The answer could not be more unequivocal: "the true philosopher despises them." The body, according to Plato, confuses the mind in its pursuit of the absolutely true. It is the cause of war when riches are acquired "because we are slaves in its service." The philosopher's soul therefore "ignores the body and becomes as far as possible independent, avoiding all physical contacts and associations as much as it can in its search for reality" (CET 5).

The *Phaedo* goes further by suggesting that not only can philosophers learn nothing from the body but that it actively leads them astray (CET 25). "The body intrudes once more into our investigations," says Socrates, "interrupting, disturbing, distracting, and preventing us from getting a glimpse of the truth" (CET 26). Thus, within the Western notion of what is appropriate for the philosopher to seek—Beauty, Wisdom, Truth, the Eternal, etc.—the body (and all that the body demands to keep functioning) is an obstruction to a disembodied Reality greatly more desirable than, and superior to, the all-too-present burdens that rest upon us now. Curtin notes drily that one response to the paradox that reality is too real has been the invention of "philosophical themes . . . to reassure us that we are not utterly temporal beings" (CET 8). For all our efforts at transcendence, however, the body's unwelcome and untimely irruptions remind us that existence mostly consists of what T. S. Eliot in "East Coker" calls "flesh, fur, and faeces, / Bone of man and beast."

Western philosophical and Gnostic traditions are not alone in their squeamishness about, and even scourging of, the flesh. (Indeed, vegetarianism in both East and West has for millennia been inextricably intertwined with the belief that meat consumption encourages all manner of carnality—lust, gluttony, and violence among them.) Renunciates within Asian traditions meditate on the body's demands, decay, and disintegration and honor the soul that's no longer bound to the cycle of karma and reincarnation. The Daoist quest for immortality involved overcoming the body's limitations through spiritual disciplines, ingesting toxic substances, and alchemical transformation.

The conviction that metaphysical existence is more real, and thus more valuable, permanent, and desirable than physical reality—and commensurately that seekers of wisdom properly direct their attention outwards and upwards to the abstract and the spiritual and away from the particular and the concrete—has had immeasurable consequences for our perceptions of the body and its functions. In her piece in Cooking, Eating, Thinking, writes Curtin, Susan Bordo "regards anorexia nervosa and other eating disorders as the psychopathological crystallization of culture, a process she explains partly in terms of the effects of Cartesian philosophy on popular culture" (CET 7). In other words, our somatophobia (the term is feminist philosopher Elizabeth Spelman's) is a concentration of a sickness that pervades Western civilization: the body politic that hates itself; that seeks to discipline it, alter it, or purge it in order to perfect or purify it.

The assumption that the body is merely, to use Descartes' term, *res extensa*—a mechanized appendage of no significance to the immortal soul or the thinking Self except in that it veils the True—has not only affected how we see ourselves, but our relationship with other animals and their bodies. Curtin comments: "A culture that defines the body as an evil impediment that blocks the struggle to realize our full human potential is deeply invested in thinking of (other!) animals as contemptible, and as unworthy of moral consideration." He continues: "commitment to vegetarianism as a healthy way of living in relation to others is a kind of 'bodily knowledge' that presupposes a process of experience in order for it to be compelling" (CET 131). To become aware of our and others' bodies as subjects to be honored and not objects to be controlled or consumed is thus a radical reframing of the Self, its boundaries, and its ethical obligations.[1]

So much, for the moment, on the (dis)connection between the

---

[1] I am indebted here to the work of Carol J. Adams and other feminist theoreticians for these observations, and for the word somatophobia (see *Animals and Women: Feminist Theoretical Explorations*, edited by Carol J. Adams and Josephine Donovan, Durham, N.C.: Duke University Press, 1995, p. 2).

body and thinking. What about thinking and moving that body? Lisa Heldke notes (CET 205) that the intellectual is supposedly disinterested, a Subject reflecting on an Object, not swayed by labor or other activity from the important business of thinking. To contemplate another requires a fixed relationship, with the separation marking a defined space. Thinking, therefore, is at risk when sidetracked by (e)motion, or other people, or moving parts; it requires isolation and stillness. The Buddha attains Enlightenment meditating beneath the Bodhi tree. Jesus retreats into the desert or up the mountain to pray. Rodin's *penseur* sits . . . alone.

Yet plenty of philosophers have been walkers: Immanuel Kant spent an hour each day in perambulations around Königsberg, and Aristotle was reputed to lecture while moving around, thus (perhaps apocryphally) the name of his school, The Peripatetics. The Danish existentialist Søren Kierkegaard unpacked the dichotomy of thought and motion in typically conflicted fashion in a letter to his niece Henrietta Lund in 1847: "I have walked myself into my best thoughts and I know of no thought so burdensome that one cannot walk away from it . . . but by sitting still, and the more one sits still, the closer one comes to feeling ill. . . . If one just keeps on walking everything will be all right." Here, movement is an escape from thoughts as much as a stimulation of them: a way of both concentrating the mind and emptying it.

Running, of course, is more intensively physical and intentional than walking. As physician George Sheehan in his work and the writers gathered in the anthology *Running & Philosophy* (R&P) observe in their various ways, long-distance running requires the cultivation of what many philosophers and moralists would consider virtues—self-discipline, tenacity, passion, consistency, drive, fortitude—as well as the power of the will, self-actualization, and even a sense of play. Sheehan believes running offers more than simply character development. It's a peak moment, akin to a religious experience: "When I run . . . the body and spirit become one. Running becomes prayer and praise and applause for me and my creator" (R&P 28, 31).

By contrast, Japanese author Haruki Murakami, a ludic writer with an unassuming, even divagatory prose style, resists making any large claims about knowledge or illumination through running: "I just run. I run in a void. Or maybe I should put it the other way: I run in order to *acquire* a void" (Murakami 17). Murakami's thought processes are unattached and evanescent, as in Zen meditation or in a state of *sunyata* (emptiness). Unlike Sheehan's, Murakami's self is evaded, even erased, through running: the *anatman* (or "not-self") to Sheehan's cosmic soul or *atman*.

Both Sheehan and Murakami are driven individuals, and yet the reasons for their dogged pursuit of running remain elusive, even to them. Perhaps it's because running is inherently paradoxical: unusual and yet quotidian; agonizing and yet stimulating; a means of delaying the inevitable decay of the human body and yet a pointed reminder of its failing powers. As runners we train ourselves to listen to the body's complaints but resist its blandishments just enough so we can keep going. What T. S. Eliot in another context calls "the movement of pain that is painless and motionless" ("The Dry Salvages") exemplifies the further contradictions: that the sore legs, blisters, shattered quads, shin splints, etc. demonstrate the effort necessary to achieve that which without pain wouldn't be possible; that we run to experience those moments when the body is sufficiently trained that we no longer give in to that pain, or when motion is so easy that it doesn't feel like we're moving at all.

These paradoxes apply to mind–body dualism itself. As J. Jeremy Wisnewski writes: "[W]hen I stopped trying to control my bodily movement with thought and concentration, I found that I was able to run freely, and moreover, to *think* freely—unimpeded by worries of how much more I would need to go before I could finally stop. My thinking did not allow me to run; my running allowed me to think" (R&P, 40, italics in original). Yet Wisnewski states in the very next sentence: "I was not, of course, always successful in this. In fact, I often failed. I often found myself concentrating on distance and minutes; on exhaustion and sweat" (41).

A philosophy of running, therefore, veers from the existential and the ecstatic to the mundane and effortful, the timeless to the time-bound, the transcendent to the visceral—even as we struggle to summon up the virtues that will carry us through to the end. Running allows us to contemplate nature through the seasons and the passages of life, or even observe the brother- and sisterhood of runners who, like us, follow the familiar paths and byways each morning. Yet running's regular beats (the ticking of the race clock, the split times as the miles add up, one's pulse, the *pflap pflap pflap* of one's shoes on the ground, and our inevitable decline through the years) all point to the temporality that Curtin observes so discomforts some aspects of the philosophical endeavor, and yet which consume the runner. (Eliot's "Burnt Norton" suggests another relevant paradox: "Only through time time is conquered.") Even when we discover ourselves in a moment out of time (the body moving effortlessly through space, the sunrise at the top of the hill) we're inevitably drawn into the placement of the next step and the next breath. Running's being is unavoidably committed to its becoming.

The lack of a settled philosophical outlook is, I would suggest, inherent in running's discourse (*discursus*: "a running from one place to another," or even "a runaround" [R&P xi]). We never land in the same place twice. And that digressiveness might be necessary, because to make any larger claims about our running experience is inevitably to draw attention to our physical insufficiencies. Grounded in the experiential and particular, running is relentlessly situational: our mood and training regimen, the course, the weather, the time of day, how fit mentally and physically we feel that morning. Every definition degrades or is surpassed (*gradus* and *passus* both mean "a step" in Latin), whether up, down, or straight ahead. Running leans in to the *flexus*: the turn, the swerve, the transition. Not every run is epiphanic; some excursions are embedded in discomfort and self-loathing, journeys into one's inadequacies. That's why, for me, we're on surer philosophical ground when we think about running as deflection or inflection, a glance or hint, the cadence and accidence of stress, the pressure and load and the spring and lift from the foot.

Of course, this anthology is not merely concerned with eating and walking/running, but *veganism* and running. Why rarify or intensify the argument to this extent? One reason to employ veganism and running as tropes is to focus an argument on what we might conceive of as the appropriate definition of what food and the animal *are*, and thence the "correct" relationship one might have with their, and our, bodies. Another reason is to place deliberately and deliberatively before us the *conscious* process within the everyday actions of consuming food and propelling one's body. Because veganism and running are willed processes, they bring to the fore the thinking that occurs (or doesn't appear to occur) in what most of us would consider automatic actions, such as walking and eating.

Yet, when we talk about veganism and running, can we be sure of what we mean, and do they really have anything to say to *each other* about what it means to be human or the conduct of a good life? This volume not only wagers that they do but offers an initial outline of Curtin's hope for *Cooking, Eating, Thinking*: that it will suggest "various ways of approaching that subject matter."

WHEN I READ Curtin and Heldke's work in 1993, I remember how unusual it seemed that a book would treat food as a locus of political and social import, let alone philosophical discussion. Shortly after graduation, and partly influenced by the pieces in *Cooking, Eating, Thinking*, I became a vegan.

A year later, in 1994, I cofounded a magazine, *Satya*, which brought together ideas and reports on activism in the environmental, animal advocacy, vegetarian, and social justice movements. Five years after that, I began a publishing company, Lantern Books, which explored the same themes, often from a religious perspective. In creating these venues for the written word, it was my belief that apparently disparate and even ostensibly opposed movements to generate change in our relationship with the biosphere held more values and ideas in common than they were willing to countenance. I still feel that way. My work since has focused on weaving these strands of thinking together.

My decision to adopt a vegan diet was largely a result of my concern for the rights of nonhuman animals and my worries about environmental degradation. Yet it was already clear to me in 1993 that not all animal advocates were vegans and not all vegans were animal advocates—however much one subgroup might wish it of the other. Indeed, the term *vegan* was controversial: some used it only to refer to their diet (free of milk, dairy, and meat, but not necessarily of honey); others took it to also mean not wearing wool, silk, or leather; still others avoided all animal products (including the above, and casein, lactose, gelatin, cochineal, and other "natural" additives made from animal's bodies). For some, veganism was a regimen to reduce the risk of heart disease and certain cancers, with an emphasis on clean living and fitness, and little stated interest in animal rights or welfare, let alone pollution, social justice, or food security. For others, veganism was all about other-than-human beings, and what you put into your body (no matter how processed or chemically enhanced or dubious its provenance) didn't matter as long as it contained no animal products.

Twenty years ago, I recall that vegetarianism's role models tended to be those blessed with brainpower and moral conscience (Mahatma Gandhi, Leonardo da Vinci, Leo Tolstoy, etc.) rather than physical prowess, perhaps because most of us weren't engaged in athletic activities. Animal rights and vegetarian groups continued to court celebrities, some of whom were involved in sports: tennis legend Martina Navratilova, Olympic track star Carl Lewis, and wrestler "Killer" Kowalski were among the favorites in the 1980s and 1990s; Peter Singer in *Cooking, Eating, Thinking* mentions Finnish middle-distance champion Paavo Nurmi, basketball star

Bill Walton, "Ironman" triathlete Dave Scott, and Olympic hurdler Edwin Moses (CET 188).

In evoking the names of athletes whom we'd heard had once expressed an interest in vegetarianism or were reputed to be eating a plant-based diet, we vegans were attempting (a little desperately perhaps) to conscript a force that could compete against the advanced weaponry of Meat and its metaphors. Vegetarians and vegans, we averred, could be as strong and energetic, competitive and forceful, and as physically accomplished as meat-eaters. Nor, we hastened to add, did vegetarianism and veganism entail a life of scarcity and thrift, asceticism or self-denial: no need to wear a dhoti, eat mung beans, chant "om," or, for that matter, commit yourself to any political or liberationist cause, animal or otherwise. One could be as gluttonous and venal as any meat-eater, as excessive or unhealthy as any gourmand dedicated to consuming animal muscle. As if to prove that the more things change, the more you can remain the same, food scientists over the last two decades have come closer and closer to replicating the creamy fatness of dairy and the sinewy chewiness of flesh—the "mouth-feel," as they say in the trade—in their fake meats, faux milks, and ersatz cheeses.

Part of me looks at the growth of interest in veganism in the two decades since the publication of *Cooking, Eating, Thinking* with wonder. Non-dairy milks and meat analogues are ubiquitous in supermarkets throughout North America. Most restaurants serve vegan options, and many more establishments are solely vegan. The word itself has moved from being misunderstood or sneered at as the diet of cranks, misfits, and health nuts to the center of the plate: the Eden from which consumers can take their solitary way to find the amount of "sinful" meat and dairy acceptable for their fallen lifestyle.

Another part of me, however, scans the good news and wonders whether veganism hasn't lost something radical and antinomian as it's been subsumed into consumer culture and become for some a personal choice associated with reversing heart disease, regaining sexual potency, losing weight, looking younger, or simply being trendy. I admit my demurral might be a reluctance to concede that veganism has evolved into all that we could realistically hope it to be—or, more subversively, what it perhaps always was: merely another diet and lifestyle choice among many; an omnivorous majority's accommodation for the tiny subset of people who maintain the regimen, for whatever reason, on a more-or-less regular basis.

Here, too, *Cooking, Eating, Thinking* has proved instructive. The book was published at the outset of a resurgence of interest in how and what we eat: the efflorescence of the Slow Food movement, organic farming, locavorism, Community Supported Agriculture, community gardens, greenmarkets, and artisanal baking and brewing. Since then, a number of books have paid critical attention to factory farming, fast food, monocultures, the alliance of biotechnology with agribusiness, and chronic obesity throughout the industrialized world and, now, within developing nations.[2]

---

[2] For instance, here is a sample of books questioning meat-based economic and health policy from 2013 to April 2014: *Meatonomics: How the Rigged Economics of Meat and Dairy Make You Consume Too Much—and How to Eat Better, Live Longer, and Spend Smarter* by David Robinson Simon (San Francisco: Conari, 2013); *Food Choice and Sustainability: Why Buying Local, Eating Less Meat, and Taking Baby Steps Won't Work* by Dr. Richard Oppenlander

Yet reading Curtin and Heldke's anthology again after twenty years, one is struck by how many of the issues raised in the book have yet to be addressed seriously in public policy itself. Cash and commodity crops are still being grown and traded at the expense of food security around the world. Varied food cultures continue to vanish amid the international consolidation, homogenization, and corporatization of the production, distribution, and consumption of food. And climate change (then newly popularized by Bill McKibben's *The End of Nature* in 1989 and Al Gore's *Earth in the Balance*, published in the same year as Curtin and Heldke's anthology, and at the time largely a theoretical and not present danger), is now threatening human and biotic communities throughout the planet.

The emergence of "foodism" as a very visible manifestation of the lifestyle and identity of upper-middle-class white urbanites can all too easily disguise for the *bien pensant* among us the continued challenge many other Americans face finding fresh natural produce at affordable prices to feed their families. Although published when Earth's population (as the book notes) was four billion, *Cooking, Eating, Thinking*'s admonishments about the need for food justice have in general yet to be heeded or acted upon. The severe consequences of the globalization of industrial animal agriculture for

---

(Minneapolis: Langdon Street Press, 2013); *Whole: Rethinking the Science of Nutrition* by T. Colin Campbell (Dallas: BenBella Books, 2013); *Food Over Medicine: The Conversation that Could Save Your Life* by Pamela A. Popper and Glen Merzer (Dallas: BenBella Books, 2013); *Farmageddon: The True Cost of Cheap Meat* by Philip Lymbery and Isabel Oakeshott (London: Bloomsbury, 2014).

food security, health services, and climate change (let alone animal welfare) have yet to register in the corridors of power.[3] One shudders to imagine what readers will make of this anthology twenty years hence, when the global population will have doubled since the early 1990s and Earth's ecosystems are even more compromised, perhaps unrecoverably so.

That a volume could still appear so timely after two decades is a testament to Curtin and Heldke's remarkable prescience. It's also a depressing reminder of how difficult it is to shift from those liberal bromides we consumers tell ourselves about how market forces can bring about change and how what one eats is *only* a personal choice—when what is needed is seismic, systemic reorganization if all are to be fed healthfully *and* the planet's bioregions protected. *Cooking, Eating, Thinking*'s commitment to the notion, expressed in many of its pieces, that in addition to the philosophy behind French cuisine or the Zen of cooking rice, "thinking" about food necessitates a re-examination of sociopolitical and cultural norms, gender relations, and economic disparities, remains a deeply radical act.

Running, too, faces dilemmas about its identity. In 2007, I decided to take up long-distance running (something I write about in *Lifelong Running*, a book I co-authored with the pioneering vegan athlete Ruth Heidrich). Perhaps it was because I was finally paying attention, or perhaps because a genuine trend was emerging, but I noticed that vegans and vegetarians were becoming more interested

---

[3] The public policy "action" tank Brighter Green (www.brightergreen.org) has produced a number of papers on the effects of industrialized animal agriculture on climate change and other issues.

in endurance events, such as marathons, ultramarathons, and triathlons.

And it wasn't just ordinary also-rans such as myself. Superstars like Scott Jurek (winner of the Badwater Ultramarathon, Spartathlon, and the Western States 100-Mile Endurance Run multiple times), Brendan Brazier (winner of the Canadian 50-km Ultramarathon Championships in 2003 and 2006), Rich Roll (who completed five Ironman triathlons in seven days), raw vegan Tim van Orden, and Ruth Heidrich herself (who has won hundreds of races over many decades) were competitive with or even outperforming their omnivorous peers. More significantly, they claimed that their diet was not incidental but integral to their success.

That running and veganism can complement each other is exemplified by Mike Fremont, who in April 2013 completed the Knoxville half-marathon a few seconds shy of three hours and four minutes. What made this otherwise decidedly unremarkable feat noteworthy was that Mr. Fremont was ninety-one years old when he crossed the finish line, and his time was a world record for men of that age.[4] Fremont, who took up running relatively late in life, didn't credit his performance only to training. He told *Running Times'* Mike Tymn, "When you get to be my age, you're not going to be able to train at all unless your body holds up. I simply cannot overemphasize the importance of the plant-based diet to my perfor-

---

[4] "Mike Fremont, 91, Finished Knoxville Half Marathon," by Michelle Hamilton, *Runner's World*, April 8, 2013. See <http://www.runnersworld.com/races/mike-fremont-91-finishes-knoxville-half-marathon-304> (all URLs accessed March 24, 2014). See also Heidrich and Rowe, *Lifelong Running*, pp. 104–5.

mance." In addition to eating no meat or dairy products, Fremont also took no supplements or medication, and in twenty years of maintaining a whole-foods vegan diet he'd not gotten sick at all.[5]

Mike Fremont wasn't, and isn't, unique. In 2013, vegetarian athlete Fauja Singh retired from competitive running, which given that he'd turned 101 years old was understandable. Since taking up running again in 1989 after a gap of sixty years, he'd accomplished a great deal—including, when he was a hundred, shattering eight world age-group records in one day.

Vegetarians and vegans aren't only present in sports that require endurance. In 2013, Patrik Baboumian walked ten meters with more than half a ton of weights on his shoulders: a new world record. After yelling "Vegan Power," he then added that his aim had been "to inspire people and break stereotypes that tough guys need to eat a lot of meat." That same year, fifteen vegan body-builders, competing at a tournament under the team name "Plant Built," came first in five of the seven divisions, and another member ranked in the top four.[6] I recall jokingly telling friends that it was no longer enough of a challenge for vegans to stay moderately healthy, as had been the case in the 1990s. Nowadays, one had to be a super-successful athlete and/or power-lifter to prove that one was fitter, stronger, bigger, and badder than every omnivore.

Since 1992, distance running has like veganism moved from the

---

[5] "Eat Right. Paddle. Run Easy," by Mike Tymn, *Running Times*, April 8, 2013. See <http://www.runnersworld.com/masters-profiles/eat-right-paddle-run-easy>.

[6] "Vegan Bodybuilders Dominate TX Competition," by Melissa Nguyen, *VegNews*, August 3, 2013.

periphery into the mainstream of American consciousness—at least rhetorically and disproportionally, given that the Centers for Disease Control reported in 2013 that only twenty percent of adults in the U.S. exercise adequately, let alone run, and that only half a percent of Americans have ever run a marathon.[7] In the year that *Cooking, Eating, Thinking* was published, 28,000 people competed in the New York City Marathon. In 2013, there were 50,304 finishers.

Nowhere has running's newfound popularity been more in evidence than with the Boston Marathon—a race for which you have to qualify unless you're running for charity or you're invited by the organizers to take part. In 2008, registration for the event, which is run in April, closed in February of that year. In 2009, all the places were filled by the previous November. In 2010, the entire race was sold out within *eight hours* of registration opening in October, which precipitated a staggered application schedule for the 2011 race (a situation that obtains to this day).[8]

Not only has participation increased since 1992, but so have the number of races. According to C. J. Schexnayder, organizers in the U.S. and Canada in 2012 staged more than 720 marathons

---

[7] "CDC: 80 Percent of American Adults Don't Get Recommended Exercise," by Ryan Jaslow, CBS News, May 3, 2013 <http://www.cbsnews.com/news/cdc-80-percent-of-american-adults-dont-get-recommended-exercise/>, and Marathon Running Statistics <http://www.statisticbrain.com/marathon-running-statistics/>.

[8] Blog post: "5 Reasons Why the Boston Marathon Sold Out in 8 Hours," DC Rainmaker, October 20, 2010. See <http://www.dcrainmaker.com/2010/10/5-reasons-why-boston-marathon-sold-out.html>.

(only about 300 marathons were run in 2000), with "the number of U.S. marathons topping a thousand finishers" more than doubling between 1999 and 2011. Schexnayder observes that the huge growth in participation in marathons has likewise meant an increase in the training miles run by those competitors: "Running USA's survey of 11,800 runners found that US marathoners ran approximately 4.4 days per week for an average of 29.4 miles."[9]

"Ultras" (any run over 26.2 miles), triathlons, and Ironman competitions (a 2.4-mile swim, 112-mile bike ride, and then a marathon), which used to be the domain of only the most dedicated of entrants, are now more popular than ever[10]—as are assault-course-type races ("tough mudders"), where participants wade through mud, scramble underneath barbed wire, and leap through hoops of fire (among other indignities).

It's perhaps no coincidence that, just as old-fashioned vegans like myself may lament what we perceive as the diminishment in political engagement and/or commitment to an encompassing vision of our diet beyond personal well-being, so some hard-core runners feel discomfort at the popularization, even bastardization of their sport over the last twenty years, as it becomes more corporate, commercialized, and commodified.[11]

---

[9] "The Marathon More Popular than Ever," by C. J. Schexnayder. Stridenation.com, February 28, 2012. See <http://www.stridenation.com/2012/2/28/2830407/the-marathon-more-popular-than-ever>.

[10] "Ultramarathons Gaining in Popularity," by Josh Tapper. *Toronto Star*, June 16, 2012. See <http://www.thestar.com/sports/2012/06/16/ultramarathons_gaining_in_popularity.html>.

[11] This lament is a thread throughout Christopher McDougall's bestselling

As I argue in *Lifelong Running*, running has helped many people become fitter, rediscover discipline and purpose in their lives, and raise a lot of money for worthy causes. But the surge in interest has also been accompanied by slower average times for men and women, a refocusing not on winning or competition but in taking part and personal growth, and even a dialing down of discomfort and difficulty in favor of expending no more energy or time than necessary to cross the line and get your medal and other swag.[12]

The fabled loneliness, idiosyncrasy, and even misanthropy that used to define the long-distance runner have been replaced by friendly, charitable packs of runners trundling through large cities, and spending money on colorful costumes, expensive watches, and all manner of paraphernalia. And gender plays a role in this perception. Running used to be the domain of maverick men, and perhaps acquired the identity that male philosophers like to apportion to themselves: that of the fearless individual stretching his mind and body beyond the bounds of the known. Now, particularly in half-marathons, more women than men take part, and the races have taken on a more collective identity.[13]

Born to Run: A Hidden Tribe, Superathletes, and the Greatest Race the World Has Never Seen (New York: Vintage, 2011).

[12] For example, the comments expressed in "The Slowest Generation" by Kevin Helliker, *Wall Street Journal*, September 19, 2013 <http://online.wsj.com/news/articles/SB10001424127887324807704579085084130007974>.

[13] Gina Kolata discusses the thorny issue of women's competitiveness across age groups in "See Jane Run. See Her Run Faster and Faster," *New York Times*, August 30, 2007 <http://www.nytimes.com/2007/08/30/health/nutrition/30Fitness.html?_r=0>.

In making these observations, it behooves us once more to reflect on the legacy of *Cooking, Eating, Thinking*. Like the earlier anthology, we, the contributors to *Running, Eating, Thinking*, are compelled to recognize that we're fortunate in ways we might, quite literally, never imagine. The tens of thousands of us who pay the hefty entrance fee, buy the tech shirts and expensive shoes, and set our fancy watches and snap our "selfies" at the outset of the race, may find it hard to appreciate the extraordinary personal dedication of the athletes from East Africa who more often than not finish the races we enter one, two, or three hours ahead of us.

We may put the remarkable achievements of the Kenyans who dominate the races down to the high altitudes of their training camps in the Rift Valley or the supposedly special genetic gifts of the Kalenjin ethnic group they tend to come from. But we rarely consider that the very limited economic options for these men and women make running a highly desirable way of earning a living, which thus encourages fierce competition, and that the excellence reinforces the desirability of being the best. Nor do we take into account how, as children, they're obliged to run six to ten miles each way to school each day because of poor infrastructure and the remoteness of their settlements.[14]

We runners would also do well to recognize that more than a quarter of Americans are obese (defined as possessing a body mass index of over 30)[15]—a chronic condition that has numerous negative

---

[14] One runner who does is Adharanand Finn (see bibliography).

[15] See "U.S. Obesity Rate Rising in 2013," Gallup Well Being, November 1, 2013 <http://www.gallup.com/poll/165671/obesity-rate-climbing-2013.aspx>.

effects on health and that could be treated by creating more opportunities and incentives to move your body. The magazines and blogs we read are filled with inspiring stories of individuals who recovered from life-threatening illness or lost weight by changing their diet or taking up running. Yet the decline of manufacturing jobs, a sedentary lifestyle, and infrastructure that favors the car and not the pedestrian point to the need for a systemic reinvention of the workplace, conurbations, and rural areas if *large-scale* health improvements are to occur.

Likewise, we vegans by choice should remind ourselves that some people are too poor to purchase animal protein; that they inhabit locations with few options to acquire fresh fruits, vegetables, and other whole foods; and don't eat enough of anything, let alone a healthful diet. As much as we may assert, with some justification, that our regimen would be cheaper and more readily available if inequities and imbalances in the global food distribution system didn't make it easier to produce and deliver low-quality or highly processed carbohydrates, sugars, and fats than whole foods and grains, our privilege cannot be brushed away as incidental. Can those migrant workers who pluck our fruits, harvest our nuts and seeds, and pick our vegetables afford the abundant produce they make available to us and which we buy with such little thought?

Nor, frankly, do we runners retain top of mind the sacrifices and challenges faced by those unable to run at all. Although wheelchair and handcycle races now allow disabled athletes to compete and earn prize money, and prostheses provide amputees with increased mobility and the chance to participate fully, it would be a mistake to assume that all those who wish to move can now do so. We easily forget that our supposedly "free" sport depends on access to parks, sidewalks, and safe neighborhoods, as well as the leisure time to be able to squeeze in a run.

Our speculations about running or veganism, therefore, come laden with perhaps unspoken or unrecognized class, regional, and economic privileges that need to be voiced, at the very least. That we might not think these realities affect our thinking is to reveal a prejudice as old as philosophy itself. Attendant on the various luminaries at Agathon's drinking party in Plato's *Symposium* are the slaves who gather, prepare, and deliver the food. Unlike the guests, the servants cannot afford to neglect the things of the body in their feeding of these minds.

These very rough, even coarse outlines of the trajectories of running and veganism over the last two decades demonstrate that veganism and running remain contested questions. Are they merely lifestyles that anyone can partake of without necessarily loading them with any greater meaning than a personal choice to become fitter and eat more healthily? Or do they—or more pointedly, *should* they—challenge our preconceptions about our abilities and our responsibilities toward ourselves, others, and the planet that sustains us? And if the latter, then who gets to determine what those responsibilities entail?

One might resist the latter implications by pointing out that one can be perfectly fit without being a runner and a superb runner without being a vegan. You can be a model citizen and care deeply about the world without being either vegan or a runner. In fact, some runners appear to resent the notion that their activity might be anybody else's business but their own.

Anyone who visited the social media sites of New York Road Runners in the immediate aftermath of Superstorm Sandy in 2012 (which tardily led to the canceling of the New York City Marathon that year), or *Runner's World* when the magazine ran a story about how Texas state representative Wendy Davis wore Mizuno running shoes when she was filibustering an anti-abortion bill,[16] or read the comments attached to the video of President Obama and Vice-President Biden running in the White House as part of Michelle Obama's "Let's Move" campaign,[17] will find abundant proof that runners don't possess any coherent ideology, are no kinder to one of their own or others than anyone else, and react strongly against what they see as the politicization of *their* sport.

Likewise, you can comb the biographies of the vegan super-athletes we've mentioned and discover only the briefest mention of protecting the environment or honoring the rights of animals on their pages. Some, like Scott Jurek, who was an avid hunter as a youth, are eager to emphasize how little they feel they can comment on such matters. In their writings, these vegans extol the virtues of their diet because it helps them perform to the best of their ability—no more, no less.

------

[16] See "Filibustering Texas Senator Has a Runner's Endurance," by Jon Marcus, *Runner's World*, June 26, 2013. See <http://www.runnersworld.com/general-interest/filibustering-texas-senator-has-a-runners-endurance>.

[17] "Obama, Biden Run for 'Let's Move," by Hannah McGoldrick, *Runner's World*, February 28, 2014. See <http://www.runnersworld.com/general-interest/obama-biden-run-for-lets-move>.

WITH THESE OBSERVATIONS in mind, and considering the loose definitions of "veganism" and "long-distance running," how might we outline some philosophical linkages between veganism and running?

The first, and most obvious, connection is that both are fully embodied activities. It could be the case that personal circumstances—a food allergy or physical disability—make it impossible for you to be vegan or, more concretely, to run. In which case, the examination of either would have a theoretical cast. Yet for the great majority of us, it's hard to be interested enough to think about veganism and running and remain merely theoretical: we'd want to know what either *feels* like. Both are grounded in the body and its needs for sustenance and movement, which, as we've seen, may make them classically "anti-philosophical," not least because the body as Socrates complains, interrupts, disturbs, distracts, and intrudes—deconstructing theory with the need for B_{12} supplements and the messy praxis of glycogen depletion, gastric distress, blackened toenails, salt deprivation, bleeding nipples, chafing, cramping, sweat, and spit.

When the body insists on its right to exist—through nourishment and movement (or when either or both are denied)—the mind is forced to recognize its dependence. Indeed, as a friend of mine discovered when he blacked out from dehydration only a mile or so from the finish of a marathon, should the body's needs not be adequately met, it protects itself and the workings of the brain by ceasing all non-essential activities, such as moving one's limbs. Stories such as this demonstrate how the body insists on reminding us of how non-peripheral it is, and, as such, how no philosophical nut can be cracked without coming to terms with the shell. As Curtin observes, acknowledging mental and physical symbiosis can lead us to recognize that other animal bodies might also express philosophical consideration (in both senses of the word), however we might label what they do "instinct" and not "thought."

The second most clearly identifiable connection between running and veganism is that both call to mind—perhaps more to their detractors than their practitioners—a discipline that can appear intimidating, Spartan, even anhedonic and anti-social. They seem extreme: "unnatural" deprivations of our instinct not to push our bodies too far; and/or private, singular activities that isolate you from others who don't share your passion or commitment. In being practices that appear to reject the straightforward pleasures of rest and relaxation, fatness, fullness, creaminess, and simple commensality, veganism and running might be considered mistaken endeavors to purge the body of impurities and excess and hold off its inexorable deterioration through a damaging regime of self-denial.

One doesn't have to read far into literature about running, or running and veganism, to observe these tropes. The mind and body need to be disciplined—the body to be trained to extend its limits, not least through harnessing the power of plants. The aim is to transform the body into a space where it no longer craves the path of least resistance, because it no longer recognizes the limitation: the boundaries of the possible have been extended; the practice is no longer a conscious choice but a way of being in the world. The psychomachia here involves stilling the appetite or the monkey mind—with its distractions, negativity, and lack of focus—through concentrating on the capabilities and sapience of the body itself. Here, we might say, Kierkegaard's wish to let go of thought parallels the disciplining of the mind found in Tibetan Buddhist lama Sakyong Mipham's practice (detailed in his book *Running with the Mind of Meditation*).

Obviously, one can be a vegan and have an unwholesome body image and diet. One can run excessively and maintain an obsessive fitness routine. Yet the same could be said for any potentially addictive or pathological activity. Let us consider a third connection, therefore; one that reverses the notions behind the second. Far from being quixotic attempts to resist our inevitable mortality, veganism and running are innate to us. Once they learn to walk, children need no excuse to run, goes the argument. All children are born vegans, and one of their first experiences of disassociation is when they have to reconcile their interest in, and love of, animals with the realization that they're eating them.

Running and veganism, therefore, are not willed impositions upon, or resistance to, the inevitable trajectory of our life, but a return to a state of Rousseauesque naturalness, unfussiness, and thus goodness. They defer immediate contentment and convenience for long-term goals: training for a race, for instance, or the hope that one day one's principles will be adopted by others and cruelty toward animals will stop. But that doesn't mean they don't offer pleasures along the way. Thus, we might imagine the essence of the human as not so much a flight from the natural as a transformation of it, or even the evocation of a deeper naturalness lost to us as we grow into our fearful, self-justifying mor(t)ality. Under this schema, the animals are likewise themselves naturalized and returned to a kind of innocence, or as symbols of strength, endurance, courage, even spirit. For instance, Sakyong Mipham describes the levels of training of the mind and body by evoking the powers of the lion, tiger, dragon, and windhorse.

In its faith in a rediscovery of prelapsarian essentials, this way of thinking is essentially metaphysical, even eschatological. Runners and vegans often use the language of conversion to describe their journey: how running and/or veganism have turned them into a better self, or restored them to a truer self, or remodeled them into a newer self. Each story has a "before" and an "after" and, often, a "moment"—the realization when all that happened before no longer obtains for the new world that lies ahead. The path opens up, the road clears, the way forward reveals itself. That such experiences are often accompanied by dramatic weight loss or by recovery from physical illness tie running and veganism inevitably to Socrates' ancient assumptions: that the body's infatuation with the pleasures of the flesh—excess, sloth, greed, venality, consumption—must be curtailed, controlled, or disciplined if a more *real* You is to reveal itself, a You capable of responding fully to the revelation you've been afforded.

As *Cooking, Eating, Thinking* so effectively displayed two decades ago, the philosophies surrounding the needs and desires of the body are varied and contradictory. This overview of some of the similarities between running and veganism demonstrates that thinking about either involves not merely reflection on what constitutes "the good life" (causing least harm, finding as much enjoyment for oneself as possible, letting no possible experience go untried) but measurements of the life itself. Is it better to aim for a long life lived moderately, or undergo riskier activities in a shorter, more intense existence? Are the pleasures ceded in fact pleasurable and can the penalties incurred or challenges undertaken not become pleasures themselves? At what point do the satisfactions of a discipline and achievement tip into obsession and self-abnegation? And are both, in fact, not deeply Platonic efforts to control the body in search of a deeper truth that lies beyond the quotidian suffering of the incarnate animal?

These questions may be essentially unanswerable. Yet if one thinks of "the good life" as less about *happiness* and more about *pursuit*, then running and ethical veganism can open up subtler satisfactions, if not solutions, for addressing the human condition. For the vast majority of us, running is not about being the best, or even the best relative to one's age, sex, region, or municipality. To be a runner is to learn one's capabilities and limits, to train one's mind and body to achieve goals, and experience pleasures that had once seemed beyond reach. To be an ethical vegan is to walk through the world at once aware of the enormous and invisible suffering of animals and yet to continue on one's path, while recognizing the limits of one's ability to create change.

As such, running and veganism offer an existential expression of our being in the world. For all that we may train and push ourselves to the maximum, age will catch up with us and we'll slow down and eventually stop. Veganism remains a gesture of protest against cruelty, even as animal products surround us in our medicines, infrastructure, and other everyday items. Yet we continue both because they reflect the value to be gained in the pursuit: the constant choosing of the absurd and principled over the convenient and comfortable.

If this sounds a grandiloquent, even self-congratulatory position to take on running and veganism, then I won't deny that both pursuits can lead to self-righteousness, even a scolding Puritanism or, potentially, a quasi-fascism as one seeks to cleanse oneself of the impurities of the flesh. What should save either from such potential dangers is humility. Unless you're blessed with extraordinary talent, employ world-class coaches, and have the time, the chances of you becoming an elite runner are next to nothing (irrespective of your possessing the financial means or supportive family necessary to make such a commitment). Likewise, for all our hopes for a more compassionate world, veganism—even if practiced conscientiously—remains an impossible goal amid the embedded exploitation of nonhuman animals. Yet each meal and each run, runners and vegans have the option of committing ourselves to the fragility and resilience of our own lives and bodies, and those of other animals, too. This is my wager, and it's the bet of the contributors to this anthology as well.

AS I INDICATED at the beginning of this introduction, *Running, Eating, Thinking* is partly a homage to *Cooking, Eating, Thinking*. What I hadn't realized until I returned to the volume is that the anthology itself is a nod to Martin Heidegger's essay "Building, Dwelling, Thinking," which was first published in 1951. This lineage, I believe, is held together by more than a fondness for present participles but by a conviction that ordinary activities reveal something about what it means to be here, and alive, and to bear the weight of philosophical attention. In fact, the lineage presents the perhaps startling possibility that it is precisely *because* these activities seem so reflexive, automatic, even autonomic, and conceptually *un*-considered and *physical*, that they reveal to us a state of being-human more authentic than any claims we might make about our *meta*physical nature.

Although a lineage expresses continuity and draws upon the common threads that tie the generations together, it doesn't necessarily remain static. Heidegger's essay is, as its title suggests, interested in what it means to inhabit a space, and how we invest spaces with meaning depending on what purpose we assign to them. Heidegger locates the parts of speech of the German word "to be" (*sein*)—i.e. *ich bin, du bist* ("I am," "you are")—in *bauen* ("to dwell"), arguing that "to be a human being means to be on the earth as a mortal. It means to dwell." The writers in *Running, Eating, Thinking* agree with Heidegger about our embodiedness, but suggest that being human means that we *move*—and that wish for movement ties us into our animality, within which we all dwell.[18]

---

[18] It's impossible, even irresponsible, to talk about a lineage of vegetarianism and animals and ignore Heidegger's association with the Third Reich: especially when we consider Nazi notions of ridding the body politic of racial impurities, mongrelization, and life unworthy of life; Hitler's supposed vegetarianism and his "love" of animals; Leni Riefenstahl's fetishization of the (Aryan) body in her film *Olympia*; and the confinement and slaughter that characterized the concentration camps. When *Lebensraum* is commandeered at the expense of others, especially those such as Jews and gypsies, whom Nazism considered to be *unheimlich*—or disturbing, irruptive, and un-homelike, with its echoes of Socrates' contempt for the body and the need for its rejection—then notions of dwelling likewise are shadowed by the ghosts of those removed so dwelling might be built. Consciousness of the other, therefore, is essential, if genuine dwelling—the mutual reciprocity of shared space and an understanding that we all have animal bodies that are our dwellings—is to be honored. For more, see *Animals and the Third Reich* by Boria Sax (New York: Continuum, 2000), *Eternal Treblinka: Our Treatment of Animals and the Holocaust* by Charles Patterson (New York: Lantern

In the concluding segment to his "Building, Dwelling, Thinking," Heidegger links the building—which connects spaces in its interior and divides them in its separation of inside from outside—to *technē*, the Greek word that "means neither art nor handicraft but rather: to make something appear, within what is present." In other words, the technique of building is to allow the experience of dwelling, which has nothing to do with the building *per se*, to open up through the space that is created by the building. Until this happens, the dwelling place remains invisible to us. Heidegger's inversions evoke his concept of *Lichtung*, the clearing in the forest, shaped by the absence of trees but taking on the presence of dwelling by its capacity to reveal to us the hidden.

We runners like to talk about "form," by which we mean honing a technique that allows us to run with maximal efficiency and minimal drag. The notion is that through approximating a correct form, one can, paradoxically, leave the form behind and run "naturally." Of course, because we're humans and our bodies are all uniquely shaped, perfect form is impossible: we pronate or supinate; strike on the heels of our feet and not the balls; overstride or swing our arms across our chest. Even the greatest runners have to "overcome" the deficiencies of their techniques: Paula Radcliffe, three-time winner of the New York City and London marathons and the

---

Books, 2002), and "Heidegger's Hitler Problem Is Worse Than We Thought," by Rebecca Schuman, *Slate*, March 10, 2014 <http://www.slate.com/blogs/browbeat/2014/03/10/heidegger_and_the_nazis_the_black_notebooks_suggest_he_was_anti_semitic.html>. Shadowing my discussion of animals and Nazism, Western anti-Semitism, notions of purgation, expulsion, and the hatred of the body is Sander Gilman's revelatory *The Jew's Body* (London: Routledge, 1991).

women's world-record-holder over the distance, bobbed her head as she ran. We remind ourselves to keep our form. Yet, who hasn't run in the hope that at some point the technique is honed enough that it falls away to leave us dwelling in the opening that is pure running?

We look at the gait of the cheetah or the lope of the wolf with envy: how fluid and effortless it seems! Might we also hope that running has the potential to reveal to us the animal that has been hidden in the meat or dairy that we eat? The animal is of course present within the transformation that becomes meat, and yet is veiled by language and the removal of the *anima* that gives us its presence. The revelation—the opening up of Heidegger's clearing—is that the embodied creature that wanted to run and was unable to do so is the same as us: no less fleshly, no less mortal, no less straitened by their inability to stretch their limbs, and no less perfectly imperfect. At that point of connection, the techniques of running and veganism (the building) can fall away to reveal the joy of movement and the identity of non-harming (the dwelling) that, paradoxically, has no singular body and is contained by no skeleton. In sum, the building of the physical reveals the dwelling of the metaphysical.

It's in the spirit of this relay, then, that we pass the baton of finding our space and eating and thinking on from Heidegger through the contributors to *Cooking, Eating, Thinking*, to the vegan runners of this anthology. The book is divided into three sections, each reflecting the slightly different orientations of the vegan runners who contributed. Befitting the thesis behind this approach to philosophy, each piece is grounded in the occasional harsh reality of lived and embodied experience: attempts to conquer ill-health and sickness; recognitions of the confinement and bodily constraints of other-than-human animals; and the joy we all share at being alive in the open air.

It's possible that in twenty years what's written here will seem either dated or prescient, or both—another step in the long run to a greater understanding of what the great race of life is about. In the meantime, however, it seems only appropriate, given Heidegger's settlement on *bauen*, to dwell, and its neighbor, *bauer*, the farmer, that the opening chapter should be by Gene Baur, the creator of the safe space for domesticated food animals that is Farm Sanctuary!

Brooklyn, NY
March 2014

RUNNING

1

A Marathon, Not a Sprint

Gene Baur

I've always tried to keep in shape. Although I was neither a serious runner nor did I sign up for races when I attended high school and college in Southern California, I would run frequently behind my parents' house in the Hollywood Hills. In my last year of college at the University of Rhode Island I was on the cross-country team, but I spent most of my time playing Ultimate Frisbee! Before I co-founded Farm Sanctuary in 1986, I hitchhiked around the country and sometimes ran up to ten miles through the cities that I stopped at. I found it a wonderful way to get to know a place: to trace its parks, visit its monuments and sites, and locate the vegetarian restaurants.

I've only taken up running marathons and training for Ironman competitions in the last few years, inspired by vegan athletes like Brendan Brazier, Scott Jurek, and Rich Roll. For some years, I'd wanted to push and challenge myself. My father had undergone a heart attack in 1997 and a year later had walked the Los Angeles Marathon. I was inspired by his effort, which got me thinking more about running a full marathon. During Farm Sanctuary's campaign to ban sow gestation crates in Florida in 2000–02, I found myself running more than usual—sometimes eighteen miles around Watkins Glen, the home of our East Coast sanctuary in upstate New York. But I wasn't systematic about my runs. I wore old running shoes and a raggedy cotton T-shirt, and on some of those long runs I didn't drink any water. Not surprisingly, I became dehydrated and felt terrible, and this inhibited me from training properly.

As I approached the end of my fifth decade, I decided that it was time to take my efforts to keep fit and well to a new level, and to be more disciplined and serious about it. A Farm Sanctuary member and runner named Tatiana Frietas, who knew I was interested in pushing myself more, started to email me notices about upcoming races. It turned out that one of them, the Oak Tree Half-Marathon, was due to take place not far from Farm Sanctuary, in Geneseo, New York. I signed up to run and on September 5, 2009, I finished in a time of 1:40:34. My running friends told me that this time was a solid indicator that I was in good enough shape to run a marathon in a time between three-and-a-half and four hours. I was intrigued at the prospect, but didn't pursue the endeavor immediately. After completing a couple of shorter races in 2010, I finally bit the bullet and signed up for the Rock 'n' Roll Marathon on March 17, 2012, in Washington, D.C., where I'd recently relocated and met my girlfriend, who is a triathlete.

Even though I'd trained more intently than previously, including a couple of twenty-mile runs, I assumed that I would finish within the time frame indicated by my 2010 half-marathon. Following other runners' advice, I started out slowly, because I was worried about hitting "the Wall" and what might happen to me at mile twenty. At mile 18 I felt so good that I pushed on and finished in a time of 3:28:03. On this occasion, I made sure that I drank properly throughout the race!

Since the Rock 'n' Roll Marathon, I've moved on to do triathlons, including a half-Ironman, and two more marathons—including the 2013 Los Angeles Marathon, which I completed in a personal record of 3:22:58. In July 2013 I completed the Lake Placid Ironman triathlon in just under twelve hours. I've even been profiled on the "I'm a Runner" page of *Runner's World* magazine.

THESE ARE THE statistics about my running career, short as it is. But I'm not that interested in detailing those achievements—even though it's satisfying to be able to show people that you can be a middle-aged man, a healthy vegan, *and* take part in the toughest races, thereby helping to dispel the myth that vegan food is somehow lacking in nutrition or that we need animal protein to be able to compete.

More importantly, running has shown me a way I can clear my head and process ideas. It enables me to work with the questions that trouble me (and everyone else) at Farm Sanctuary: What strategies should we adopt to bring an end to a particular form of animal exploitation? What should be our next legislative push? How can we go beyond or reconcile the arguments regarding animal welfare and animal rights that continue to plague the animal advocacy movement?

Instead of stewing over these issues indoors or at a desk, I lace up my shoes and head out the door. Running not only allows me to burn off excess negative energy but also lets whatever's going on inside me bubble up to the surface in a way that I'd describe as "detoxifying." In other words, the constancy of my inhalation and exhalation as I take to the trails not only seems to even out my heartbeat but extracts the anxiety or emotional baggage from a concern that's been weighing on me. I find myself able to examine the problem with a degree of equanimity and objectivity that, I believe, makes it easier to solve, or at least view from differing perspectives and with a proportional response. Running gives me the space to go through various scenarios, assessing the pros and cons, and try to figure what will or won't work.

But there's a deeper connection that keeps me going. In running and breathing and exploring the world through the physical body that was given to me, I'm connected to the most fundamental expression of our animal nature. In my almost thirty years with Farm Sanctuary, I've campaigned to educate people about the obscene conditions under which the animals we raise to eat live and die. I've visited stockyards and factory farms and witnessed horrendous abuse and neglect, which I've documented in photographs and on videotape. I've seen animals who are unable to turn around in their cages or stalls; who've been fed a mineral- and vitamin-deficient diet and are too weak to stand; who can't move because they're chained, or confined in factory-farm warehouses, or abandoned on "dead piles" when they were still alive, with dead or dying animals piled on top of them. I've come across cows and sheep and pigs so sick that they've collapsed in the stockyard ("downers") and have had to be dragged or forklifted onto the truck that will take them to the slaughterhouse, or whipped and electrically shocked onto the chute that will lead them to their death.

Farm Sanctuary's response has been to promote veganism; to ban the worst factory-farming cruelties, including gestation crates, veal crates, and battery cages through legislation and popular referenda; and to end the misery of the downers by legally mandating proper medical attention so they don't suffer any more than they have to.

But even those animals who aren't victims of special cruelty suffer in our modern industrial food system. Many of those who are fortunate to make it to Farm Sanctuary because we've rescued them from stockyards, farms, slaughterhouses, or from accidents on the highways, have been genetically manipulated in profound and disturbing ways. Turkeys, for instance, should be able to fly and roost in trees, but because we have bred them to produce the largest amount of meat possible, these birds grow so fast and large that they can barely walk, let alone fly. They have been so fundamentally altered that they cannot even reproduce naturally; they all have to be artificially inseminated.

My everyday experience over the last three decades has been to bear witness to how completely factory farming and the culture that supports it deny other animals the simple pleasures of moving their bodies in a way that they want to. The nineteenth-century German philosopher Arthur Schopenhauer is reputed to have said, "We are what we eat." It's a maxim that has never seemed truer than today. Just as the obese and immobile animals whom we raise for food are full of drugs to make them grow fast and because they're so chronically unhealthful, so we as a nation are more and more resembling the creatures we consume.

Farm Sanctuary offers a respite from the horrors of industrial animal agriculture. I've observed more times than I can recall how a calf or a piglet who arrives at the farm starts for the first time to run around, kicking up her hindquarters and expressing sheer joy and exuberance at being alive. I've seen how avidly they relish the fresh air instead of the noxious ammonia fumes of a chicken shed; how they enjoy letting their hooves sink into the soft grass instead of slamming against metal grates or concrete floors; how quickly they start to flap their wings or dustbathe or wallow in mud for the first time—all acts unavailable to them on factory farms. These creatures may have lived every moment of their short lives in a barren cage no bigger than their bodies, but when given the opportunity to express who they *are*, even the most genetically manipulated of them want *to try* to move. It's a transformational experience for both the animals and the people watching them.

At Farm Sanctuary we've been honored to become the home for animals who've exemplified this fundamental wish to be free in the most literal manner possible: they've run away from their places of confinement. Queenie, a five-hundred-pound cow, escaped one day from a meat market in Queens, New York. After running through the streets, she was eventually captured by the police. She became an instant media celebrity and we finally persuaded the city and the slaughterhouse, whose property Queenie was, to let her live out the rest of her days at Farm Sanctuary.

We may want to think that Queenie is exceptional and that the many billions of other sentient creatures who are killed every year in the United States for food have less desire to live. Queenie *was* smart in that she saw an opportunity to flee and literally ran for her life. But she's exactly the same as all the other animals. They hear the screams, smell the blood, see the blade or the bolt, and feel rough hands taking them to their end. They know the terror of being yanked off their feet, or drowned and scalded. In fact, because many of those we eat for food are prey animals, they're especially sensitive and alert to threats to their lives. It's not that they don't want to escape; they've been programmed to run. They simply can't. Denying these creatures an ability to move only exacerbates their panic and shock.

After seeing how these animals behave when given the chance to *be* animals and not machines, it's evident to me that movement is not merely a function of our being animals, it's an expression of *self-identity.* None of us can truly be ourselves unless we're free to move our legs, or breathe in and out through our lungs, or shake our arms or wings. If we're denied the ability to move, we become depressed and defeated, and ultimately we won't flourish. We may even lose the will to live. This is as true for me as it is for a chicken, turkey, pig, goat, sheep, cow, or any other animal that we throw inside a cage until they're killed—or discarded on the dead pile because they're of no use to us.

Of course, I'm not saying that all animals (human or nonhuman) who are born with disabilities or who lose a limb aren't capable of leading fulfilled and happy lives. Indeed, animal sanctuaries across the United States continue to welcome many animals who have required the amputation of their limbs or are otherwise handicapped because they were neglected or abused. We provide them with the prostheses they need and the medical care they deserve, and they enjoy the shelter, love, and care of our staff, members, and volunteers.

AS AN ANIMAL advocate for farmed animals of many decades, I know very well how dispiriting it can be to be a voice for those whom so many people only think of as sources of food—if they think of them at all. Running has not only allowed me to blow off steam, but has made me aware of how our work on behalf of these creatures is a marathon and not a sprint. Our work requires discipline, persistence, and patience. Working at Farm Sanctuary and training for these punishing distances have made me appreciate how vital it is to remember the saying attributed to the Daoist philosopher Laozi: "A journey of a thousand miles begins with a single step." We can sit at the starting line and discuss strategy about which would be the right way to run. But, in the end, a marathon is always 26.2 miles and to reach the finish you have to take the first step, and then cover every yard of it.

We may fret over the immediate controversies, irritations, and setbacks that make it seem as though we're making little or no progress and exhausting ourselves in the interim. But our work—our race—demands that we focus on short and long-term goals, and ultimately get across the finish line. At the same time, we realize that it will never be attained unless we start changing our diets, educating ourselves about the terrible reality for billions of farmed animals, and speaking out on their behalf.

I'm now over fifty years old and I see no reason to slow down.

In fact, I want to grow stronger and be more effective in my activism and my running, and other activities too, like swimming and biking. I'm pleased to say that I've gained more energy from my fitness regimen and a diet that's clean, green, and empowering. They enable me to continue my work to free all those other animal bodies who don't have the luxury of feeling the sun and the wind on their faces, breathing fresh air, and stretching their limbs. It's my hope that, eventually, we'll not just survive together, but thrive.

2

Running Is Compassion

Colleen Patrick-Goudreau

I was once asked in an interview how running affects my being vegan and how my being vegan affects my running. That's like asking how breathing affects my being alive and how being alive affects my breathing. There simply isn't a place where one ends and the other begins. They are intricately linked.

I imagine the answer is different for people who came to plant-based eating to improve their health and even to improve athletic performance. I'm encouraged by the number of runners and professional athletes who are eschewing animal-based meat and animal products in order to be faster and stronger and experience more endurance. And certainly a diet based on whole plant foods will garner those results.

I came to veganism through a different door. I was raised in a typical American family eating the typical American fare: anything that walked, swam, or flew. Veal Parmesan was a common menu item in our house, Chicken á la King was my favorite dish, and

I drank chocolate (cow's) milk with abandon. I didn't necessarily choose these foods. They were chosen for me. Nobody told me what they were made from, and when I asked, my parents and the adults around me either evaded the question entirely or deceived me completely.

I was also typical in that I cared very deeply about animals. I loved being around them, I had no fear of them, and I intervened and wept whenever I saw them suffering. I don't think I loved animals more than most children do, and my parents and the adults around me supported and encouraged this compassion in every way. Images of baby animals adorned all of my clothing, wallpaper, and bedding; animal cut-outs hung over my crib in a musical mobile; and stuffed animals were my constant companions in and out of my bed. I sang songs about animals and played games where I mimicked animals; I was brought to the zoo to admire animals; and on many a Halloween, I dressed up as an animal. More than that, animals were used to teach me my most fundamental skills through characters in books and television shows who showed me how to count, how to spell, how to read, and how to talk. Through the use of myths and fables, animals even taught me such values as respect and kindness, and I learned social mores through their teachings.

In every aspect of my life, I was given the message that nonhuman animals were integral to who I was, even shaping who I was becoming. But what I didn't know (because nobody told me) is that I was being fed the dismembered bodies of animals—the very same animals I was brought to the zoo to pet. The very same animals whose wings I helped mend. The very same animals whose faces were depicted on my pajamas.

And so I was taught—implicitly, of course—to categorize animals into arbitrary and paradoxical compartments of those we love and those we eat, those we live with and those we exploit, those worthy of our compassion and those undeserving of it because they happen to be of a particular species or bred for a particular use. In other words: puppies good, calves food.

At the same time, I was also learning to compartmentalize and temper my compassion. I was given the message that life is not always fair and nature is not always kind but that God put animals on the earth for us to eat and that I should be grateful for His kindness and their sacrifice. That fierce, unconditional compassion I had as a child began to become dulled, as my taste for animal flesh and fat began to grow and settle into my palate.

Luckily, when I was nineteen or twenty years old, I picked up *Diet for a New America* by John Robbins, and the course of my life changed forever. This was the first book to examine the effects of our animal-based diet on our health, on the environment, and on the animals themselves, and it was certainly the first time I had ever seen the images of animal factories, where lives are regarded as machines and the value of the animals determined only by what they produce. I stared at photos of hens in cages with the tips of their beaks seared off, female "breeding" pigs confined in crates the size of their own overgrown bodies, turkeys packed in windowless sheds, calves chained to boxes. I remember staring at those images in utter shock. How could I not have known about this? How could I have contributed to it? How could this even happen? I knew I didn't want to be part of it, so I stopped eating land animals that very day.

I liken this experience to an awakening, because the lens through which I saw the world changed completely, and the compassion I had known as a child became quickened in my heart. It wasn't simply that I had come to learn something new; it was more that what I had always known in my heart had become uncovered—fully revealed. A veil was lifted, and I was awakened to my true compassion. I "became vegan."

I'm struck by how funny that phrase can sound. We say a caterpillar "becomes" a butterfly or a seed "becomes" a flower and can easily imagine what they look like in their transformation. But what does it look like to "become vegan"? Indeed, the idea that eating vegetables rather than animal products can be likened to a metamorphosis might sound strange, but that's exactly what it was for me. Through this awakening, I stepped into my authentic self. Although I had considered myself a compassionate person prior to becoming vegan, that compassion had been dulled in favor of conforming to the status quo notions of which animals our society values and which animals we have the right to exploit and consume. I had been practicing selective compassion. "Becoming vegan" was my metamorphosis into embracing my unconditional, unfettered, unabashed compassion, and it was as natural and effortless as the process is for a caterpillar becoming a butterfly or a seed becoming a flower.

THE COMPASSION I live by applies not only to how I treat and perceive others; it also applies to how I treat and perceive myself. And so, I became a runner.

Unlike the ease of my vegan transformation, becoming a runner took effort, perseverance, time, and discipline. In fact, I hated running when I first began. All my adult life I've been involved in some form of intentional exercise, and for a long time, cycling was my passion, both as a means of fitness and of transportation. In the same silly way as we choose one form of exercise over another (the way we peg someone a "dog person" or a "cat person"), I scoffed at the idea of running, proclaiming that it was too boring. I declared, with no actual evidence, that it was bad for your knees and back. I happily categorized myself as a cyclist and a hiker, both of which enabled me to spend ample time out of doors, which I've always loved. (Hence, my move to California as soon as I finished graduate school.) Nature is my church and where I find peace, and though I do prefer indoor plumbing to outhouses, I've been hitting the hiking trails since I was a wee lass.

Hiking became my single form of exercise when cycling ceased to be. This was a conscious decision borne out of fear (and pain) after a bike accident left me wary of riding on city streets. While pedaling home from the YMCA one day several years ago, I was "doored," riding in the designated bike lane. I must have blinked for a nanosecond, because I never saw the truck door fly open. I only knew that I hit what felt like a concrete wall and went flying off my bike and into oncoming traffic. I must have lost consciousness for a moment, because it took me some time to understand what was happening. The driver of the car that had almost hit me was helping me out of the street and onto the curb, and I couldn't identify where all the pain was coming from—my throbbing arm? My cut-up hip?

Luckily, I escaped with only a broken elbow and mangled bike, but once I recovered and my bike was repaired, I just couldn't bring myself to ride again. Riding was a means of transportation for me but, living in a city, I had no choice but to ride among cars and trucks, and I was just afraid of doing so again. As I wasn't an off-road rider—I'd rather walk wooded trails than ride them—I hung up my bike and eventually sold it, though it still breaks my heart to say so. The first and last time I got on a bike since that accident was several years ago when my husband, David, and I were visiting Block Island, a resort off of Rhode Island that is virtually car-free.

I continued going to the gym but, living in California, it just felt artificial. I began to hike more regularly in the forests not far from my home, but it didn't provide the challenge I sought. I still do hike once or twice a week—but I wasn't satisfied with it as my primary form of exercise; frankly, I just never felt like it afforded me a proper sweat-inducing workout. I bought a used stationary bike, but it confined me indoors. And so, I began to run.

At the time, David and I lived within walking distance of a collegiate jogging track, and we would run a few miles together each week. The track itself was probably about a quarter-mile around, so we'd run in several circles before even hitting a mile. Then two. Then three. Just as I had feared: Boring! More than that, David and I would run together—pretty much at the same pace—and as we ran next to one another, I felt bad about having my ears plugged with my iPod earbuds. It just felt rude. So, I forsook listening to anything while we ran, and as we went round and round in circles, I was left to my own thoughts. No music for rhythm. No lectures for edutainment. Just as I had feared: Boring!

I ran, but I hated it. I didn't own it. I did it because it got me outside, it enabled me to burn more calories than when I hiked (within the time frame I allotted myself for daily exercise), and it was convenient to walk out the door and hit the track. I considered going back to a gym, but the idea of paying to work out inside when I lived in one of the most beautiful parts of the world was unappealing. And so I ran—and was bored to tears.

Then, one day, everything changed. David was bending over to tie his shoe on the way to work, and his back went out. He was laid up for a bit, then he was nursing it by avoiding running, and he eventually had back surgery. In the meantime, I lost my running partner. Though David later recovered completely and started running again, that time was just what I needed to save me from my running ennui.

Unconstrained by someone else's running schedule, preferences, and pace, I was compelled to create my own routine. Without David to talk to, I created a playlist on my iPod, and with a preference for running on the neighborhood streets rather than on a small track, I literally hit the pavement. I felt liberated. That's not to say that my husband is or was a hindrance in any way, but if we were running together, I felt obligated to run at his pace and on his terms and thus made myself feel constrained. David never imposed this on me; it was all self-inflicted, and I didn't even realize I was letting myself experience constraint—until it stopped.

I bought a Garmin watch, I upgraded my running shoes, and I began creating a running route—first a couple miles in a loop staying close to home, then venturing farther afield, beyond my immediate neighborhood. As I began to run longer and farther, I even had to expand my playlist, as I began to outrun the length of songs initially chosen. Nick Cave and The National joined Midnight Oil and Clap Your Hands Say Yeah in motivating me on what became four-mile, then five-mile, then six-mile runs. (Of course, a number of songs from my husband's band, Gosta Berling, graced my playlist from the beginning, so David was running with me after all!)

Music propelled me forward and helped me create a running rhythm, so I never understood when people would tell me they listened to the vegan podcast I produce (called "Food for Thought") while running. I couldn't imagine running to spoken words rather than music. Eventually, that changed, too. And now, though I would never say I will never return to music once in awhile, podcasts now dominate my listening pleasure. The audiobook of Stephen Mitchell's translation of Laozi's *Daodejing* was my gateway, and now I use my runs to listen to Public Radio Exchange's *The Moth*, Chicago Public Media's *This American Life*, and the hundreds of university lectures offered by The Great Courses that I never had time to listen to before.

And so, while I can't put my finger on the exact moment, at some point during this time I became hooked. I became a runner. Prior to that, I was someone who ran. I did it because it was an obvious, convenient form of exercise, but I hadn't owned it. It wasn't mine. I did it despite the fact that I didn't enjoy it.

I knew I was becoming a runner when I found myself planning my days around my runs, when I began logging my time and distance, and when I began subscribing to *Runner's World* magazine. But the day I really felt it, the day I truly stepped into my running self, was the first time I ran in the rain. Prior to that, I had often felt disappointed when the forecast called for rain, because it meant I couldn't run, but the day I said, "Rain be damned! I'm running anyway" was when I knew something had shifted. I felt so strong, so powerful, and so proud, and that day I stopped seeing our beloved Northern California winter rains as a hindrance to my running. I had become a runner.

By the time David recovered from his surgery, I was fully obsessed, and I began urging him to join me. But this time, I had no qualms about running ahead or running with my earbuds—and of course, he didn't either. He was cautious about returning to the track, and it wasn't until the surgeon told him that he could have gone running months before that David started up again. He ran mostly on the track and around campus but would sometimes join me on the street. The neighborhood we lived in then was very hilly, and though I don't love running on hills, I experienced many blessings while running on those streets. Because my veganism/consciousness/compassion accompanies me wherever I go, it turned out that running has afforded many opportunities for animal advocacy and provided many gifts in return.

On a crisp March day, on one of my daily runs, I had the pleasure of meeting a little cat named Charlie. Although I do truly stop to greet any animal who will grace me with his or her presence, if he or she is a tuxedo cat, I simply plotz. All of the cats I've intentionally adopted have been black and white tuxedos, and Charlie was no exception. I'm a total sucker for tuxedo cats. It's not just how cute they are in their formal attire, it's that they're part dog/part cat. I can't explain this, but if you ask anyone who's ever lived with a tuxedo cat, they'll tell you the same thing. They're incredibly social (after all, they're already dressed for parties), inquisitive, vocal, and extremely smart.

When I saw this adorable little kitty lounging on the sidewalk, I knelt down to say "hi," and before I knew it, he jumped up on my leg and put his two paws on each of my shoulders. Of course, I fell in love immediately. I saw him several times after that on my daily runs (and took David down to meet him), so one day I decided to knock on the door of the people I had a feeling he belonged to. Indeed, he had been newly rescued from a neglectful and border-line abusive situation, and the couple had taken him in along with another abandoned kitty, whom they hadn't realized was pregnant. So now they had Charlie, this other kitty, four new kittens, their own kitty of many years, and six small dogs. Well, I told Charlie's guardian that I adored him (by now she had witnessed this herself, as well as Charlie's mutual affection for me). She asked if I wanted to adopt him since he was not getting the attention he deserved. We had lost our cat Simon the year before; the timing was right, and we made Charlie part of our family.

Although I very consciously allowed this situation to turn into an adoption, this is just one of the many times I've encountered animals on my runs. Most of the time, it's just a matter of greeting them, but sometimes I've had to stop my run completely to provide aid, and luckily these situations have always resulted in happy endings: a dog I returned to his yard after he wandered out of his unlatched gate; another dog who had jumped over his fence and escaped into the street and needed to be returned to his house; a couple of rabbits who had escaped without their people's knowledge—a quick knock on the door resulting in the rabbits being brought back inside; a homeless cat whom I brought to the shelter (and who subsequently got adopted). None of these encounters would have occurred had I not been out running. They're among the many gifts I reap from what has become my primary form of exercise, which—incidentally—is also a gift to myself.

BECAUSE WE LIVE such sedentary lives, we tend to look at intentional exercise as a necessary evil, unless we find something we love. We exercise because we "have to" or because it's the "right thing to do." But unless a particular form of exercise gets under our skin, we perceive it as a drudgery that we have to reward ourselves for in order to stay motivated. There was a time when I thought that way, but I don't anymore. In fact, it's quite the opposite: running is the gift I give myself. Running is an act of self-compassion. Rather than feel like I deserve a treat for running, I perceive running as a treat I give myself after working hard. When I finish writing a chapter of a book, an editorial, or a podcast episode, for instance, the reward at the end of these satisfying but arduous tasks is a run.

Participating in daily exercise, eating healthful whole foods, and nurturing my spirit are very powerful reflections of self-love. Though I still add them to my daily list of goals ("run five miles," "prep veggies," "meditate"), I do them all with great enthusiasm, though not without effort. They're part of my daily routine, but I'm still very proud when I accomplish them. Habits though they are, they're also conscious acts of self-care, as are brushing and flossing my teeth, washing my face, and taking multivitamins. It's because I care about myself that I do these things, and doing them regularly means they become habits. As such, they're not optional.

Just as my compassion for animals doesn't wane, neither does my compassion for myself. There isn't a day when I think, "I don't care about animals today, so I'll eat a chicken." My compassion for animals is consistent, and so there's never a time when I want to commit violence against them. So, too, is my compassion for myself. That doesn't mean that when I don't run or eat exceptionally well that I'm reflecting self-hatred (my self-esteem isn't nearly that fragile), but it means that my default is to take care of myself, while allowing myself periodic indulgences.

One of the ways I can measure how I treat myself is when external factors intervene. Recently, I experienced an unenviable year of loss, grief, and fear due to circumstances outside of my control. One of my closest friends—who was also my assistant—died unexpectedly and tragically, and my beloved cat Schuster followed him three days later. Two months later, I was embroiled in an unjust legal issue that threatened my happiness and my work. It was an incredibly painful time, and I thought it would never end.

No one would have been surprised if I had sunk into a depression (and I was close), or medicated myself into oblivion, or retreated from the world completely. And yet, when I reflect on that year, what I'm most proud of is that I took care of myself throughout the turmoil. I continued to eat well and meditate, and I ran on a regular basis—even when I didn't want to. I wanted to crawl in a hole until it was all over, but I cared too much about myself to let that happen, and so I ran. I do not exaggerate when I say that there were days when I couldn't stop crying such that I'd be running with tears streaming down my face. (It definitely made it hard to breathe properly!) I remember one such time when I actually had to stop, kneel down on the sidewalk, and sob because I quite literally couldn't breathe for all the tears that came. A woman kindly called down from her balcony, asking if I was all right, and I told her I was. I got up, wiped my tears, and kept running.

And that's ultimately what running is for me and why it's tied into my being vegan. For me, being vegan is about being compassionate—to ourselves and others—and running is one of the ways I demonstrate compassion for myself. The rewards I reap are organically tied to the act of running: the awareness that I've done something good for myself, that I've taken care of myself, that I set a goal and followed through, that I felt powerful and strong while I ran, that I increased my endurance and learned to run faster and longer, that I experienced the joy of solitude, and that I used the time to listen to favorite podcasts and lectures.

That's not to say that I run without difficulty or discomfort. When I've experienced running-related injuries and pain in my ankles, knees, and hips, I struggle to remind myself to treat myself with the same compassion that I would treat someone else with similar injuries. I ice, I elevate, I stretch, I massage, I rest, but sometimes I push too hard before I show myself some compassion. And that's the power of running: it affords me the opportunity to demonstrate and reflect my compassion—both for myself and for others—and in doing so, I manifest what it means to be vegan in every aspect of my life.

3

The High Life

James McWilliams

At the end of a race, the legendary University of Oregon runner Steve Prefontaine would appear weirdly comatose. The muscles in his legs would strain into a million ropy fibers, but his face would turn to putty. It was like he was watching golf. This involuntary escape from otherworldly pain—the runner's high—is what every endurance athlete, professional or amateur, aims to achieve. For long-distance runners in particular, this enviable trance is not unlike yielding to a seductive drug—an elusive experience that, could you bottle it, you'd be doing most of your running to the bank.

It's natural to speak of this state of mind as a form of detachment, a lapse or an escape into an ethereal cocoon. That's not exactly the case, though. The mind and body under such circumstances aren't disengaging so much as blending in a way that's transcendent and calming. Who knows how anyone ever reaches this mystical apex? Who really grasps the inner mechanics of such an unexpected form of euphoria? I suspect that there are as many paths to this state of being as there are people fortunate enough to discover it.

For me, I learned that this kind of high could also be experienced by being vegan. In 2007, after nearly thirty-eight years, I stopped eating animals. Veganism and running, in turn, became complementary sides of my evolving identity, inseparable and mutually reinforcing phenomena that have worked me into a more whole, or at least less fragmented, person than I once was. Before veganism, running was something I did. After veganism, it was an essential part of who I'd become: a humble agent of change.

A CAVEAT: AS an athlete I'm nothing to get excited about. I'm persistent, for sure, but certainly no star. In the course of running more than twenty-five marathons and several ultramarathons, and with the benefit of almost twenty-five years of running experience, I'm in a position of doing a few useful things: I can weave my own running narratives, identify my own lessons learned, appreciate my own trips into "runner's high" transcendence, and lick my own self-inflicted wounds. I've been running almost every day for nearly two-thirds of my life; I have stories about running and, like most runners, I enjoy telling them. All that said, as a runner, I am, on a good day, an average talent.

Another caveat: While veganism was the defining hinge in my personal history as a runner, I'm in no position to proselytize (who really is?). Which is to say, I'm not suggesting that an athlete *must* go vegan to achieve any benefits. That would be crazy. And obnoxious. And possibly even counterproductive. The vast majority of addicted runners I know—and I'm talking about people who will happily scrape themselves out of bed at 4:30 A.M. to run twenty miles in eight-degree weather—are running with incisors, and they intend to use them much as their hominid ancestors did. Most runners I know rip flesh from bone with enthusiasm. Indeed, perhaps touched with a little paleofantasy, they are perfectly happy to tap into their inner caveman, chase down a feral pig, build a fire, and eat the beast without care or compunction about ethics or nutrition.

I just know that, as a runner, I can speak truth to one reality: my own. For me, running and eating plants have become not only necessarily intertwined, but mutually reinforcing and transformative endeavors that empower me to rage in the best way I can over what it means to not only live, run, and eat, but to stand up for the most vulnerable in a quest for justice. These endeavors, I've since discovered, are worth a commitment. They are worth sacrifice. How they were merged is, in many ways, the story of how I became the person I am.

MY INITIAL AWAKENING as a long-distance runner happened suddenly. It was a crisp fall late afternoon in 1988. I was in college in Washington, D.C., and had just bombed a physics exam, effectively dashing whatever slim chance I ever had of getting into medical school. I dressed up for my normal three-mile run and felt overcome emotionally—which is to say I basically felt like a loser. All my insecurities were coalescing in a dark place. Under a sky that had exploded into a kaleidoscope of blue and orange, I left the house and, on cobblestone streets, passing the townhouses of the power elite, did my standard three-mile run. Usually, my thoughts would be ironed out by the time I finished this ritualistic loop around Georgetown. But not this time. This time I remained a mess.

So I kept running. From Georgetown I headed down to the Kennedy Center, over to the Lincoln Memorial, and across the Mall to the Capitol. By then it was dark and the city sparkled. My gloominess started to lift. The simple act of moving through space in the center of a flickering city, breathing steadily, mollified me into an acceptance of a medical school–free future. I crossed the 14th Street Bridge into Virginia, ran along the parkway, cut across onto Roosevelt Island, and then headed over the Key Bridge back onto the cobblestone playground of Georgetown. Certainly, there were other vocations to pursue. I could drive a cab or be a bicycle messenger. My mind did somersaults. The coup de grace was to bolt up the famed "Exorcist Steps," a fierce Everest-like incline off M St. made famous in the unnerving 1973 horror movie I couldn't finish because it scared me so badly. But my worries were gone. Even better, I was *high*.

I guessed I'd run about seventeen miles. At home, I grabbed an icy beer and gulped it down in the hot shower. Now I was *better than high*. And I was also hooked. Over the following winter and into spring I started to explore the city's extensive trail system (Rock Creek Park), ran through parts of town I'd never explored (Hayne's Point, Capitol Hill, Arlington), and I even found a friend to do longer weekend runs with, eventually reaching into the sixteen to twenty-mile range every Saturday morning, followed by a heaping plate of eggs and sausage.

My roommates, a group of artists and writers who elevated laziness to an art form, took to calling me "Mr. Squirrel," suggesting that I was running around the woods of D.C. gathering nuts and berries for the impending winter. One friend, a painter with a special talent for inactivity, suggested that they hook me up to a generator so I could produce renewable energy. I began to shed weight. One Christmas all I received from everybody I knew was running clothes.

I ran the San Francisco Marathon in 1992. Knowing what I know now, this was a colossally stupid choice for a first marathon. Even the hills had hills. But it wasn't quite disastrous enough to ruin the idea of running marathons for good, despite the fact that I couldn't walk down stairs for two weeks after the race. Diet wasn't helping my cause. Eating at this time in my life was a remarkably passive-aggressive experience. As a young man running forty miles a week, then fifty, I'd not only eat whatever you put in front of me, I'd have seconds. And thirds. It seemed the more I ate the thinner I became. So why care? I recall looking in the mirror at my body in the basement of my D.C. home and noting that, for the first time since pre-pubescence, my ribs were poking through my torso. And I was consuming food like a Dumpster.

Essentially, to the extent that I ever pondered it, eating was an input/output experience. It was fuel. I either burned it or evacuated it. Food was functional. No more or less. This remained the case for well over a decade, and it was during this decade that my signature weakness as a marathoner became depressingly clear: I was completely useless after twenty miles. No energy. No runner's high. No transcendence. Nothing but pain.

This is a rather intractable problem for a marathoner. Not only because a marathon is 26.2 miles, but, as they say, a marathon is a twenty-mile warm-up for a 6.2 mile run. Whether on training runs or actual races, I bonked and crumbled and gorked and choked (choose your term) after twenty. Every time. And I'm not talking about discomfort. I'm talking pain that was metaphysical in nature, otherworldly, and not even worth the tears. They call it a *wall*, but that's bullshit. You can climb a wall. Or build a door into it. Or slump against it. Worse, it would take me at least ten days to feel normal again after a race.

In 2007, after a score of marathons with times that wouldn't budge, I experienced a different kind of pain. I watched a video of a calf being taken from his mother just after birth. It was one of the worst experiences of my life. How a person makes it through more than three decades without encountering such an event is a testament to the power of modern culture to sanitize the violence of reality. So I watched this clip. Then I watched it again. One more time.

As a seasoned academic (at this point I had become a historian instead of a doctor or cab driver or bike messenger) I knew I was supposed to think and deliberate and avoid reaching hasty conclusions. Indeed, I was supposed to resist sentimentality and be objective and keep a cool head. But I also knew that, as an academic, I was perfectly capable, as most academics are, of thinking myself into a drooling stupor, of having the emotional makeup of a stone, of abjectly failing to be human. So I said *no more.* In my office, I stood up, looked out the window, and literally said to myself, "No more." I thereby became a vegan with the same epiphanic concentration of conviction that I became a runner. And as with running, I've never bothered to reconsider.

———

TO ME, THE saying that life becomes a utopia after going vegan is the same sort of cheesy propaganda as "Got milk?" or "Where's the beef?" Veganism can be a big pain in the ass. Eating out becomes a small nightmare. Dinner party invitations decrease. Airports send you into crisis mode. The entire country of France looks at you funny. Your Italian grandmother thinks you're mentally ill. If a vegan tells you that it's easy being vegan, and he has anything resembling a social life or doesn't live in Vegantown, U.S.A., don't believe him. Not a word.

But, no exaggeration here, veganism saved my running. Eating a nutrient-rich plant-based diet had a remarkable impact on my post-twenty-mile dilemma. Most notably I was now regularly zooming past the twenty-mile mark feeling better than I did at mile ten. I began to do ultramarathons and was even feeling strong past thirty miles. Even more befuddling, after bombing my body with a post-run bowl of quinoa, amaranth, blueberries, cashews, and agave syrup, followed up by a banana-cocoa powder smoothie, I was recovering so quickly I could go out the next day without soreness. Recall: before veganism it would take about two weeks for my legs to feel normal. Now it was taking less than a day. So, no, life didn't become a utopia, but, for the first time, I was running daily with pure joy.

Buttressed by veganism, my running—which had resumed giving me a high—did something unpredictable and wonderfully generous. It turned around and began the long and slow process of making my personal veganism political. I began to whisper some of my ideas into print. Then I got a bit louder. Before long, I was yelling into the pages of mainstream magazines and newspapers that, to my surprise, wanted to hear what I had to say about animal rights and ethical veganism and moral consistency. In a twist that's even more wonderful and liberating, this activism began to inform my running. It was then that everything coalesced into something.

Let me try and explain this relationship. First: the running. Long-distance running—especially when you can do it in an ethereal frame of mind—is personal and political, but even more, it's transcendental. You transcend "normal" behavior as well as your own expectations. Over time, this serial transcendence plateaus at a different idea of "normal." Through this empowering process, you continually recalibrate your identity. You constantly create new conceptions of what's possible and those new conceptions become part of you and you become much more interesting to yourself than you ever were.

The key is this: You become more involved with the world as an agent of change. You rage a bit against conventions. And this entire process is modeled. Others witness it; many are pissed and jealous and hate you. But many others are moved by it—and they change for the better. In this intensifying two-step of empowerment and transcendence, you are a public model, whether you think so or not. When you start running seventy or eighty miles a week, the people around you eventually take notice and become curious about you as a person with thoughts and goals and habits. It's an exceptional thing, mainly because you're not seeking anything but inner peace. But you become a leader—ideally, a humble one.

Second: the vegan part. A very similar scenario—this internalizing, identifying, witnessing, and modeling—happens with vegan advocacy. My chances of convincing a non-runner to run by declaring "Run!" are the same as convincing a non-vegan to go vegan by declaring "Go vegan!" Basically zero. Yes, you have to make your case, and there are a million ways to do it, but ultimately you have to do so while putting yourself out there, by allowing yourself, although scared to death, to be witnessed. It's risky, and people will scream at you, but there's really no other choice if you want everything to become something.

A long-distance runner cannot hide her running identity any more easily than a vegan advocate can hide his vegan identity. Nor should they hide it. Exposure has its costs, for sure, but the rewards are sublime; just ask any ethical vegan or self-identified runner. In these ways, both long-distance running and ethical veganism etch positive standards—personal and political—into the pantheon of unrealized possibilities. To an extent, to be a vegan runner is to be the humblest of revolutionaries.

A revolutionary mentality, at its essence, demands several qualities: the ability to waver between individualism and community, the ability to not care when people you admire, love, or disagree with you (or end up hating you), the ability to choose peace over force whenever possible, and the ability to admit when you're wrong and not gloat when you're right. And, in doing all this, you will never feel more right.

I think running and veganism, when brought together, have a spiritual way of imparting and nurturing the emotional preconditions of many revolutionary-minded qualities. I won't go into precisely how for each, but I will say this: In general, running and veganism teach humility; greed for what's good; inestimable self-assurance; and a deep sense of what really matters. These attributes strike me as critical for any effective revolutionary mentality, whether collective or individual. Animals will never thrive in a human culture of arrogance and indifference.

SINCE BECOMING A vegan, I often have to stop in the middle of a run because the force of the experience overwhelms me so. It's as if you cannot be more present in the world at that moment. And the beauty is, you don't need to do anything. Just exist. And run. And not eat animals. Every distraction evaporates and you feel completely, fully alive and stunned at once.

This happened to me while running trails alone in the mountains around Eugene, Oregon—Steve Prefontaine's hometown—about three years ago. It was an impossibly crisp day. My run began in the city and, as I dealt with traffic and noise, my mind started to clutter with the data of daily life: work, bills, deadlines. I was dealing with a sore foot at the time and feeling sorry for myself as I left the city behind and entered the woods. When I hit elevation, my breathing picked up. As I reached about twelve miles, I turned a corner on the trail. Next thing I knew, out of nowhere, I was seized by the beauty of the forest around me, by the calm that fell over me, by the empowerment that characterized my life. I found myself, a vegan-ultramarathoning-revolutionary-writer-activist living the high life, leaning against a Douglas Fir tree, as hopeful and happy as I'd ever been in a world marked by pain.

4

Beating Destiny

Ellen Jaffe Jones

Recently, a Facebook running site I follow posed the question, "What are you running from?" My instant answer: "Disease!" Every time I start a race or cross the finish line, I think about disease and what it has done to my family.

My earliest childhood memory is of my aunt dying of breast cancer in our home when I was four. I remember the screaming, crying, and wailing. She was in her late thirties and left behind her daughter, my five-year-old cousin. After her death, my cousin and I would hug each other in our bedroom. I could only imagine her terror at being left without a mother at such an early age. She would rock herself to sleep many nights. On my part, I learned to be very afraid of breast cancer and to avoid it at all costs.

This set in motion a lifetime quest to dodge genes that would get my family enrolled in the research studies done by Myriad Genetics to identify and patent breast cancer genes. The odds of any female in my family getting breast cancer is 1:4. The national average is about 1:8. As an investigative reporter in my twenties, thirties, and forties, I often said that dodging breast cancer became the story of my life. From that early terrorizing moment in childhood, I began to view the world with the thought, "How do I avoid this mess?" Being the youngest of three daughters, with two sisters nine and eleven years older than me, I had many years to see what worked and what didn't work.

When I was twenty-eight, the younger of my two sisters got breast cancer for the second time. That year, I watched her deal with the ravages of chemotherapy and radiation, and held her as she vomited. Only then did I begin to understand what she and everyone else who had breast cancer at the time had to go through.

I was now the only healthy person in my family. By a long shot. But it wasn't always that way. Earlier that same year I had a colon blockage so large that the doctors in the emergency room said they had never seen anything like it. They told me I would need to be on medication the rest of my life. I knew I was way too young for that. So I ran to the health food store and read all five books on fiber that were in publication at the time.

Through books like *Don't Forget Fibre in Your Diet* by Denis Burkitt, I began to understand that my beginning stages of colon disease were from a lifetime of not eating enough fiber and not getting enough exercise. I also began to see how a blocked colon, crammed with putrefying toxins, was a likely breeding ground for the cancer that gripped our family. Later, bariatric tests showed that my colon was an extra foot longer than normal from the chronic constipation and distention as I was growing up.

As far back as elementary school, my friends made fun of my

abdominal distention, joking that I must be pregnant. I remember visiting the pediatrician several times after my family went out to eat to celebrate special occasions. My mother was sure it was appendicitis. The doctor would feel around and proclaim each time, "It's just gas." I was given laxatives routinely to help deal with my chronic constipation. One laxative that my mom kept in the refrigerator tasted like chocolate fudge. I snuck into the fridge one morning and had an extra tablespoon or two. By the afternoon, Mom had to be called to school to come scrape me out of the girls' bathroom.

My poor mother. She, like all of us, just tried to do the best she could with the sorry information that was available at the time. At that time, in the 1950s, Castoria was the laxative of choice. One ad claimed it was "better than prunes." The idea that a liquid medicine could be superior to fiber-filled prunes, a real food, seems ridiculous now.

After my colon scare and personal food epiphany, I tried to bring my sister a bag of whole grains, beans, and vegetables from the health food store. "How dare you!" she angrily said. "I've made my choice of how I want to treat my cancer. Don't undermine my decisions."

My sister, who would go on to get breast cancer a third time, often said, "It isn't a matter of if I get cancer, but when." Despite my own health issues, I vowed it would never be my turn. I would be the one to beat the odds and set out to figure out how. I swore that genes would not determine my destiny.

It wasn't just cancer that brought my family down. Here's the final disease tally on my family tree:

- *Heart disease and diabetes*: mother, father, sister, two grandparents, all aunts/uncles
- *Alzheimer's*: mother, grandmother, uncle
- *Colon disease*: Everyone. Dad had a colostomy.
- *Arthritis*: Everyone
- *Osteoporosis*: All women except one sister

I was told by my family and doctors alike: *These diseases are all genetic.* I didn't buy it. When I learned that there were African tribespeople who had as many bowel movements in a day as our family of five had in a week, I began digging for the truth about food.

I remember my sister undergoing chemo and radiation, watching her constantly retch in pain and agony. I thought, *There just has to be a better way.* I began to read more. The connection between unplugging the colon by flushing away putrefying toxins with high-fiber foods and water seemed so obvious. Anytime I thought of returning to my previous way of eating, the visual of my sister suffering popped into my consciousness.

I began changing my way of eating through a macrobiotic diet, popularized by the book *Recalled by Life* by Dr. Anthony J. Sattilaro, who said the diet reversed his own cancer. The regimen consisted of a plant-based diet with white fish, added oils, seaweed, and seasonal and locally grown produce. The macrobiotic rules were too stringent for me, a busy television reporter whose only chance at food some days was the drive-through at Taco Bell. I morphed to eating vegetarian, and then vegan.

As I often say, many people don't "get to vegan" in a straight line. It can be filled with zigzags and bumps along the way. Like many during the 1990s, I became confused by the Atkins craze. I thought the science had changed and that animal protein was healthful. What I would later realize was that only the marketing had changed, not the science.

By now the mother of three daughters, I had left television and spent five years as a socially responsible financial consultant at Smith Barney. The ratio of men to women was 10:1, and I found it challenging to maintain a plant-based diet in a world of catered mutual-fund and annuity-company client dinners. Office-funded working lunches were pizzas and subs. Labeled by my colleagues as "Earth Mother in a Suit," I chose my battles carefully.

After that, I joined my husband in his media consulting business and we moved to Florida. Six months later, at the age of fifty, I found myself in the emergency room a second time after trying to quash a three-week-long hemorrhaging period from hell. After an ultrasound, the ER doctors wanted to do a hysterectomy to remove fibroid tumors. My regular obstetrician got on the phone and said, "Ellen, go back to that plant-based diet and call me in the morning." Within three weeks, all signs of menopause were gone. I never needed the hysterectomy or any hormone-replacement therapy.

Six months later, twenty-five pounds lighter, my cholesterol had dropped from a high 203 to 154 and I was feeling in amazingly great health. I started taking up my long-abandoned passion for running. I began on nearby beach trails interspersing walking and running. It would take me a year of doing that before I got the courage to join a local running club. I would tell everyone who would run with me about how a miraculous vegan diet wiped out menopause symptoms and gave me all of this newfound energy. It would take me another year before I dared to show up at a race. My first 5Ks came in close to forty minutes. Just a few years later, after much training, my personal record was 27:50—a time faster than my best thirty years before.

A third hospital experience was instrumental in changing how I lived my life. When I was fifty-five, the older of my two sisters, the one who didn't have cancer yet, went in to the hospital for "routine" herniated disc surgery, most likely caused from a lifetime of poor eating and inactivity. She'd already had diabetes in her early twenties, when I was twelve, and heart surgery in her fifties, when I was in my late thirties and having children for the first time. With a compromised immune system going into surgery, she flatlined on the table, almost died, and came out with MRSA (methicillin-resistant Staphylococcus aureus, a bacteria that is resistant to antibiotics) that lodged in her neck.

In a cosmic irony, my sister was placed in the intensive care unit in a bed next to my father, whose diabetes, heart disease, strokes, and thirty years of smoking had caught up to him with what would be his final episode of congestive heart failure. He had been in an assisted living facility in St. Louis, Missouri, where my sisters still lived, and I had been calling every day to check up on him from my home in Florida. When I phoned on New Year's morning, the nurse told me that I'd better come home. "They took him to the hospital last night," she said. I didn't make it to my father's bedside before he died. While I had been prepared not to see him alive, I hadn't expected to also see my sister in the hospital.

The nurses had me put on a gown and leave my potentially

MRSA-carrying phone outside the room. "Since you now know that MRSA runs in your family," the nurse said, "you don't want to set your phone down on anything in the room that might be contaminated." *MRSA runs in my family?* MRSA is in the air, on the beach, and on gym equipment. As a vegan, I believed my immune system was better than that of meat eaters, but I said nothing. My nephew was at my sister's side when I walked into the room. When he saw me, he said, "Don't say anything to upset her." I just laughed.

My sister ended up paralyzed in most of her limbs. A year after she contracted MRSA, she came down with breast cancer. As the oldest sister, she had organized most of the family events. Now she will be in a nursing home for the rest of her life.

Although I had started running competitively for fun at this point, it was watching my sister's children accept her "genetic" fate that made me decide I would run in as many races as I could to show that you *do* have control over your destiny. That yes, as a vegan, you get enough calcium, protein, energy, calories, and anything else you need to run marathons. And those doctor's bills? They won't exist anymore.

My three daughters are in their twenties now and are just beginning to understand my lifelong, uphill battles with health. My parents were so sick and diseased by the time I had my children they couldn't lift them up, let alone babysit them. Because I waited late to have children, I want to be present for them in a way my parents never could. I want to enjoy a quality of life my folks could only dream about.

I've now placed in sixty-one 5K or longer races since 2006 when I started this somewhat accidental mission. I've qualified in every event I entered in the Florida International Senior Games—the 100, 200, 400, and 1500 meter races. Finishing in the top four qualifies me for Nationals. The goal has always been to finish without injury. I want to be able to keep running until I die, preferably running on the beach. I did my first marathon at fifty-eight years old, and was the fifth oldest female to finish. I'm often the oldest female at races, which is just fine.

I want my daughters to know that they can run at any age. But most of all, I want them to know that genes take a trigger. Even if one or more of them has the breast cancer gene, they can run far away from it, as I have done.

5

Running, Singing, and Being Vegan

Lisette Oropesa

WHY I SING

What does someone mean when they say "I sing" or "I run?" Do they mean they do it professionally or for recreation? Perhaps they hope to convey that they're good at the activity, or they only do it occasionally or for fun.

I've been singing since I was able to speak. I come from a musical Cuban family and singing is in the blood. When the whole family is always singing, you learn to join them and be part of the fun, or keep silent and be left out. I wasn't going to keep silent. I got a lot of praise from singing: compliments, requests, applause, approval.

I was born in the United States and brought up in Louisiana. My parents taught me you have to work for the things you want in life, and stand up for them; that they don't come without sacrifice. They knew what they were talking about, since their entire lives as immigrants were filled with hardships. They often used to say, "Your gift, your voice . . . it is God-given. It is a talent that you must not throw away. Make the most of it because that's what will please the Lord."

I developed my voice by singing in church and gaining confidence from my parents, knowing that my voice was a blessing and made me special. It was always nurtured, appreciated, loved, and praised. Developing this talent has given me a strong connection to something greater—a force of energy that sweeps through me when I make music and open my mouth to sing. Or even when I open my ears simply to listen.

I believe that this connection is available to everyone, in a variety of ways. Music causes changes in people. It affects your heart rate, your sweat glands, your brain's output of chemicals. It can make you feel warm and snuggly or agitated and rough. It can give you goosebumps. Books have been written about this phenomenon, but I don't think I need to explain it for you to understand.

As someone who creates music for a living, I might be expected to become jaded. But music never gets old. When music is second nature to you, it's impossible to enter a grocery store without analyzing the song being played over the speakers. You can't hear a performance without absorbing the details. And if you're a singer, you can't listen to anyone else sing without in some way being on that mindtrack yourself. If someone is struggling through a piece, you feel the strain in your own vocal cords. If someone is soaring with emotion, you're moved to tears through their voice. If someone's voice is ugly, you shudder; if it's beautiful, you sigh. This connection goes beyond the human touch to empathy.

Singing has always brought me happiness. It's my greatest

strength, my best friend, my steadfast go-to, as well as an instant ticket to friendship and admiration. It's also my crutch when I'm in pain or in agony when my voice isn't working.

WHY I RUN

My running life was born in the very opposite manner to my singing. I detested running with every fiber of my being. It made my side hurt, it was hard, and I couldn't breathe. I didn't understand how anyone was insane enough to call this fun, much less to subject themselves to it voluntarily. In school, I was always the last to finish the mile in P.E. class. The teacher joined us on the track for the run, and as I jogged along she power-walked past me. I remember seeing her pretty blond hair and the back of her head and her white-and-gray track suit. I was so jealous. The girls had to wait forever on the track for the one in last place (me!) to come in. I even remember my mile time: 13:56. I had a bad knee; I was overweight and slow, clumsy, and weak. I tried very hard to mask these shortcomings, but there were always girls (or gym teachers) around to discourage my efforts. For years after I finished grade school, I avoided "exercise" or anything remotely sporty out of resentment. It wasn't until my vocal talents took me to a crossroad that I decided I had to face these ancient demons.

When I finished college, I went directly into the top young artist program for opera singers in the United States, at the Metropolitan Opera in New York City. One of my superiors told me that while my voice was perfect, I needed to lose weight. I weighed 210 pounds. I had been receiving this advice since college and I was becoming tired of hearing it. I blamed everyone and everything else for my condition: my genes, my childhood, my gym teacher. But they weren't going to be the ones to make my body change. I decided to do something about it, to take the first step.

I signed up at the YMCA, bought some exercise clothes, went in alone, hopped on the elliptical machine, and copied the girl next to me. I didn't know the first thing about exercise, let alone heart rate, diet, or even what shoes I should be wearing. I exercised for fifteen minutes and then hobbled to the weight machines and attempted to figure them out. I tried them all, and the next day repeated the process. The day after that I did it again. I slowly worked my way up to twenty minutes on the cardio machine. After a week, I had lost ten pounds.

I had been attending the gym for about six months, and losing thirty pounds in the process, when the regulars started to notice that I was losing weight and began to encourage me. One woman invited me to a spinning class, and other members began to tell me they were looking forward to seeing me each day, because my diligence inspired them. I knew nothing about exercise, but I understood perseverance. Somehow the effort, persistence, and focus that kept me from even talking to anyone was exactly what spoke to others. We had a common bond. All of us were on a mission together.

A year after I started exercising regularly, I gathered the courage to get on the treadmill for the first time. It was awful. It hurt. However, I thought if I did it once a week or so, I'd become more proficient. The first time I ran two miles on the machine, I cheered aloud in the Y. One of the trainers asked me whether I'd be running for forty minutes. "Are you kidding?" I responded. "I can barely do twenty!" But his suggestion stuck in my mind and I decided that would be my goal.

In my mid-twenties, my life ran into a series of obstacles. I went through a long and difficult divorce, and a new relationship got off to a rocky start. I moved into a new apartment and began my professional career. I wasn't eating enough, getting much sleep, or exercising at all. I had lost a lot of weight but I wasn't happy. I was under a great deal of pressure at work and had to pull it together to sing. I was afraid I might fall apart at any moment. Too many things were clouding my mind and my emotions. I needed to find space to breathe and a way to process all the change.

I told my then boyfriend (now my husband) that I'd always wanted to be a better runner. It was the one thing I thought I could do anywhere, given my career now involved traveling. I thought that if I could become proficient, I'd always have some form of exercise. "I'll run with you," he said. And so we started. It was August and we had no idea it would be so hard. We were both a mess before we hit the mile mark, so we turned around and huffed it back home. However, we were determined to try again.

It took weeks for side stitches to stop occurring on each run and even more time for us to reach the first mile and turn around without stopping to walk. We read Danny Dreyer's *ChiRunning* to each other before bed every night, and this became the foundation of our running technique and practice.

Running began to become the one thing I looked forward to every other day, even though I dreaded the moment when it presented itself. I started learning to laugh at my nerves and to tell myself that this run was going to be great. Inevitably, I always felt better after completing it. I began to tell my friends, posting my mileage, and taking pictures. I finally joined some groups made up of singers and performers who were on a parallel journey to change their lifestyles.

I didn't begin running in order to lose weight or to help my career. I simply wanted to learn how to do it and was ready to put in the time to make that happen. I didn't care how fast I was, but I wanted to be proud of myself for going a certain distance, and extend it the next time. I wanted to enjoy the natural world around me, focus on my body and breathing, and spend bonding time with my husband (who runs with me every time, without fail).

We signed up for races, which brought us closer, even though we almost never talked during a run. The shared time we had allowed us to have more to say when we finished. In our runs, we'd come across birds and other animals. Over these last months, we've run past giant sequoias trees, in deserts, over mountains, around marvelous statues, through vineyards, during sunrises and sunsets, and along moonlit beaches. We've been in more romantic settings than most people see in movies!

Running has made me a better singer, and vice versa. Music at its most basic involves tension and release. The ultimate resolution of a cadence in the tonic, basal chord would not be so pleasurable if the composer hadn't resisted our wish to return to it with all his art. Harmony is rich and luscious precisely because of the preceding moments of dissonance. Music itself would be nothing without the silence that surrounds it; the exhale of the breath that produces the voice would be nothing without the silent inhalation that makes it possible.

That symbiosis between tension and release is obviously paralleled in running—the body caught between one step and the next, falling forward and maintaining balance. As when I sing, I must at some level remain conscious of my breathing, focus my brain, and control my emotions. Yet if I did only that, then I would seize up. I would produce notes but not music, sounds but not the song. To run with too much consciousness of the mechanics of placing one foot in front of the other can lead to obsessing over mileage, time, and the various aches and pains that can afflict you. The result is joylessness, fatigue, and, most probably, dropping out. This is why it's important to breathe evenly, lower the heart rate, and relax the muscles. We were born to run and sing; our task is to train ourselves to unlearn the resistance we have to doing what is natural.

To sing for hours on a stage and to run for hours on a course require stamina. Yet, far from one discipline making it hard for me to practice the other, singing and running have reinforced each other, bringing me energy and focus. Running relieves me of the stress of the pressure of performing at the highest level of my profession. Running with my husband among hundreds or thousands of anonymous others offers me a welcome contrast to a life lived literally in the spotlight, where everyone is judging my ability. Running is one of my meditation practices.

When I first started running, I would listen to music through my headphones. I didn't want to hear the discordant music of my huffing and puffing or to listen to my mind complaining about what I was putting my body through. I didn't want to deal with the dissonance and the tension, and so I blocked it out. However, slowly, I began to run without the music and, paradoxically, I finally began to hear: my breathing, the sounds of nature, the patter of my feet on the ground. I also started to listen to that inner voice. At first, I was scared to find myself alone with years of built-up frustrations about past failures, and hatred and anger at the inadequacies of my body. Yet by listening to the rhythm of my breathing, by accepting the body's own discipline—it's own wish to keep going in spite of all the abuse we heap upon it—I discovered that I could free myself from the demands of that particular voice and let the body sing.

WHY I EAT A PLANT-BASED DIET

I grew up eating everything, with parents who cooked dinner virtually every night. I used to hate the smell of onions, garlic, and bell pepper, which seemed to begin every single meal. But I loved black beans and rice, potatoes, and pork chops. I couldn't stop after just one chip or one slice of pizza, which is why I gained so much weight. In college, I started to use food to deal with the problems I was having as a lonely music student. While my vocal talent developed, my social skills dwindled, and food became my regular friend. It was only when this habit threatened my career that I decided to change.

About the time I began to run, I started to keep a food and exercise journal. I discovered that eating eggs was causing me to experience occasional indigestion and sluggishness, so I stopped buying them. It was becoming expensive to purchase quality meat, and so I struck that from my shopping list. Cheese was simply not worth the digestive havoc it caused, since it entailed having to run a mile simply to burn off the caloric content of one cube! It made sense economically to buy only plants.

What began as a financial decision became something else when I watched the documentaries *Forks over Knives*; *Vegucated*; and *Fat, Sick and Nearly Dead*—to name a few. What I learned was eye-opening. I couldn't believe how misinformed I'd been about milk being the only source of calcium or that beef was the best source of protein. I read Michael Pollan's *The Omnivore's Dilemma* and *In Defense of Food*, as well as *Thrive* by Brendan Brazier and *Becoming Raw* by Brenda Davis, Vesanto Melina, and Rynn Berry. I grew more and more interested in finding out exactly what the body needed to function properly, and what it took to grow food in this country.

I became a vegetarian, and then a year later (in September 2011) a vegan. Since becoming one-hundred-percent plant-based, I've never felt better, and my entire outlook on what it means to be alive has changed. I've also become much more aware of the conditions for animals raised for food and have found myself being forced to defend my newfound diet. I'm told that eating meat is natural, even though we no longer hunt for our food and no longer treat the animal with the degree of respect shown by indigenous cultures of the past. We no longer express thanks for the rare animal that we captured, or honor the spirit of wildness that bonded us.

That equal being has now become our slave, for whose domination and destruction we've developed an arsenal of weaponry and torture. Instead of the patience, perseverance, and discipline of hunting animals down, we trap them, fatten them, and force them to reproduce beyond their natural capacity. The animals live in filth and the flesh they deliver is nutritionally and metaphorically impoverished. What was rare and precious has become common and spoiled.

I feel that lack of freedom most acutely when I'm running. I will sometimes encounter an animal and experience that familiar mix of fear and admiration. More often than not, the animals are shy and keep their distance from us. We are not friends. Yet we are outdoors, breathing and moving. We are kindred.

We are also connected through our voices. Along with mating, singing is one of the most natural, indeed one of the most primal, of human expressions. Like laughter, it offers an outlet for emotions of every kind. We are obviously not unique in this respect and it's surely the case that the trill of the bird, the howl of the wolf, and the roar of the lion must have inspired the first humans who heard them to respond to and mimic those vocalizations in some way. We know that the earliest forms of song were invocations of the natural world: imprecations to the Divine, hymns of praise and gratitude, lamentations for the dead and suffering. From the extraordinary choruses of Native Americans to the mysteries of Gregorian plainchant, a spirit has transformed individuals and the choir of voices. In the same way that a long run can invoke a feeling of being outside our bodies and yet wholly within the experience of the heart pumping, so singing transforms our consciousness by centering us within the breath.

THE COMMON BOND

What it is that bind these three aspects of my life together? Certainly, singing, running, and being a vegan provide me with comfort, even a rush of endorphins as they activate the pleasure centers of the brain. All three give me that feeling of aliveness as well as control. For years, I'd eaten junk food—with all its chemicals, sugars, simple carbohydrates, sodium, and fats. I'd accepted being overweight and tired because I didn't have the energy to change and it was comfortable. It was all too easy for my inner voice to keep me in bed rather than get me on the road running or to eat a burger rather than spinach. Like any singer or runner, I needed to unfetter my complacent inner voice through toughening up my core—whether that was my diaphragm, my abdominal muscles, or (if you will) my deep connection to the animal body.

The result of this discipline is, paradoxically, freedom: the freedom of a voice trained to become supple, strong, and expressive; the freedom of a body that can move with purpose, pace, and pleasure; and the freedom of a conscience unburdened by the weight of all those chained and beaten animals. What combines all three is love and respect—to relish the shape and texture of a piece of music and a morsel of food, and the rhythm and measure of a song and a step.

In becoming a vegan, I also learned the extension of the power of awareness and connection to other aspects of my life—the environment, social justice, and the conservation of energy as a whole. Concentrating on the small gestures—buying food that is fairtrade, grown organically, or eating locally—enabled me to gain a certain control, note by note as it were, in a world where so much seems beyond our power.

My goals have now expanded. I'd like to run a four-hour marathon and sing the title role of Donizetti's *Lucia di Lammermoor* at the Metropolitan Opera. In the meantime, I train to run faster and sing parts such as in Nannetta in Verdi's *Falstaff*, Sophie in Massenet's *Werther*, and Konstanze in Mozart's *Abduction from the Seraglio*. I continue to learn more about healthy food choices and focus my mind on the grace and beauty of the natural world and the animals with which we share it.

EATING

6

I Run with Every Day in Me

Cassandra Greenwald

DARK DAYS

I don't want to try and convince myself how wonderful it will be to run today, because it's a dark day, a bad day, and I will run to punish myself, or, really, to absolve myself of the sins of eating. The mirror has become a reflection of everything I am not. I am not perfect. I am not smooth or taut (I am lumpy and jiggly). I press on my bones so I can feel them. My stomach seems so big. It will never, ever be flat enough.

In the world of body love and self-acceptance, I talk a good game—I tell people all the time that bodies and brains need fuel, and we can't make the world a beautiful place if we're starving ourselves or obsessing about thinness. But advice is easier to give than take.

I know a few people (only a few) who enjoy food and eat it freely. Through some combination of good genes, excellent self-esteem, and a zest for life, these people do not think about how processed their food is or if they should have skipped the brown rice. They do not constantly negotiate with their brains for permission to eat. They do not carry around a set of rules about eating so amorphous that it is impossible to nail down. These people come in all shapes and sizes, but most of all, they are vital and free.

That is not me. I am perplexed by food all the time, and I am always thinking about how the food in my mouth will settle into the fat on my body. I know it's terrible, but I'd be lying if I said anything else. This fixation, the self-flagellation, is the antithesis of feminism, of self-acceptance, of compassion. My veganism is about compassion, but I have yet to extend that same gentleness to this animal's body. Now that I'm older and wiser, my light days outnumber the dark ones, but I have been pushing this boulder uphill for as long as I can remember.

GYM DAYS

My gym teacher in grade school was named Mr. Hurt. I kid you not. He was tall and red-faced and all business. I know I wanted to make him laugh (I always want to make people laugh), but he barely smiled. He wasn't a drill sergeant, I guess, but he definitely wasn't interested in my feelings, about gym class or anything else for that matter. In those tender days before I actually identified myself as a feminist, I had the distinct impression that he didn't really like girls.

These were the neon-colored 1980s, when everyone wanted us to just say no (to drugs, to rides home from strangers who claimed to know our parents, to menacing Halloween candy crammed full of hidden razor blades). There was a lot to remember, even for us kids.

To keep us on track, the President of the United States himself had his own test of physical fitness, to make sure we were spry and trim and could continue to say no properly.

Oh, how I hated that test. Here's an image forever burned in my brain: the white cinderblock wall of the gymnasium, undulating and going fuzzy in my field of vision, as Mr. Hurt yells at me to hang on to the pull-up bar and try my hardest to bring my chin over the top. The entire class is watching behind me. Mr. Hurt has a stopwatch, and even though I can't see what it says, I know I am failing this test. Miserably failing. Sorry to let you down, President Reagan, but I guess I'm not physically fit.

It's not that I hated gym class. I kind of liked that one day a week when I got to wear comfortable clothes and could listen to the loud screech of my little sneakers on the floor. We played dodge ball, and I wasn't scarred for life (I think I actually enjoyed it). When it was too cold to go outside, we played floor hockey, which I *loved* for some reason. I was never very fast or athletic, but that game felt good. I ran like everyone else, up and down the gymnasium with a plastic stick in my hand, in pursuit of a rubber ball that stood in for a puck. When I say it like that, it sounds so pointless, but I felt so motivated to get that ball. And yet I hated running—I did. Field day, relay races, the timed mile. All of it made me feel terrified and bad about myself and slow. Definitely slow.

When I run today, I think about that younger me, the girl who couldn't do a chin-up. Who got picked last. Who was banished to the outfield. She doesn't chase me (of course not, because she hates to run), but I see her watching me. I will never forget her or ignore her. She laughs as I put on three layers to combat the wind chill. She likes the many different colors of ankle socks in my drawer. She wonders why I bother with the whole running thing, because I only go so far, and I always have to turn around and come back to where I started. She asks me, "What kind of journey is that?"

LATCHKEY DAYS

During the days of fitness tests and floor hockey, I was a latchkey kid. At a young and impressionable age, I wore my house keys on a string around my neck, tucked close during the school day, and used them to open the door to an empty house. My mom had multiple jobs and was going to graduate school, and my dad hadn't lived with us since my parents separated and got divorced when I was three. I was alone for only a few hours, barely two, I think, before my sister came home from middle school. The timespan for a couple of my favorite cartoon shows. I kind of liked it, in a way, because that collection of rooms and doors was entirely mine. I would turn on every single light in the house and the TV before opening the fridge. I had other rituals that I think I've blocked out, but I do remember the food and how good it tasted. Pepperidge Farm cinnamon-raisin bread, all swirled and sweet and doughy. Bowls of Rice Chex covered in rainbow sprinkles, with the first bites so crackly and the last so mushy and soft. A few ravioli, snuck out from underneath their blanket of tinfoil in the casserole dish, meant for dinner, but it was only a few, right? Who would notice?

Everyone noticed.

My sister said, "I can't believe you ate a whole loaf of bread."

My mom said, "You shouldn't eat ice cream after school." (It wasn't ice cream, I protested, it was cereal, but no one believed me.)

My sister said, "You ate your dinner. Now what?"

And so, food, my most comforting after-school friend, seemed to turn against me. Or it made my family turn against me. It was very confusing. I realized I was fat—I must have been, because I couldn't pass that physical-fitness test to save my life—and this was the hand of cards I was dealt. Alone with no one but food after school. What was I supposed to do? The entire family talked about my weight, in front of me and otherwise, and I knew, I *knew* it was so wrong to be the way I was, but it didn't feel like anything I could control. It just felt like me.

Everyone has a saturation point, and I don't remember the exact day I realized I hit mine, but I know it was in middle school. After being teased, insulted, comforted, cajoled, and sometimes even loved in spite of my weight, I woke up to the idea that I could change myself. I didn't have to look longingly at the girls in my class, who had pair after pair of perfect designer jeans that fit them the way jeans were supposed to (not right up underneath their boobs). I didn't have to spend my life hiding in stretch pants and huge sweaters, which were part of the trendy look but didn't make everyone else resemble a pumpkin.

The weird thing is that this is the point where you might expect me to say that I became a vegetarian. It wasn't. My memory is hormone-blurred for these years, but I do recall the day I decided to eat no more animal flesh, and I think it was long before I wanted to lose weight. It was a chilly Halloween, and my best friend and I came inside from collecting candy to a slow cooker full of pot roast.

It was warm and juicy, but as I chewed it, something felt wrong. On one level, it tasted delicious, but at the same time, I hated it. It was metallic and heavy and stringy and rich, and I decided that was that. No more meat.

It wasn't a big stretch or a colossal deal. My mom and dad both had been vegetarians or semi-vegetarians for most of my life. My sister loved London broil and dug in to whatever else my mom cooked up, but I could always take it or leave it. I never understood why everyone loved meat so much. It seemed there were so many other things that tasted much better. Pasta, for one thing. And entire loaves of cinnamon-raisin bread.

PROUD DAYS

Fourteen years of absorbing the messages of "fat = bad" and "thin = good" brought me to a place the summer before I started high school when it seemed like a wise idea to try to stop being the fat girl. I'm sort of proud of myself for making the decision, but I'm ashamed of how I executed it. I starved myself. Maybe that sounds like an exaggeration, but when I think of the food journals I kept that summer, they were not filled with food. They were a record of how little I ate.

Surprise, surprise, not eating much means you lose weight. Everyone noticed. I got so much praise from my family for losing weight. I beamed. *See?* I wanted to say. *This is the real me. The girl you can be proud of. She was always hiding in there, and now I know you love her even more.*

I started doing things that my friends did, because I could. Some of my besties joined the gymnastics team, and I did, too. I knew I wouldn't be doing aerials in the closing floor routine to bring home the win, but I started to embrace the idea that I could exercise and test my new body a little. When a lot of the team joined winter track to stay in shape, I followed.

Winter track was no walk in the park. It wasn't even a run in the park. Winter track meant staying for hours after school, running in the halls and going through an endless gauntlet of circuits that involved wall squats and sit-ups and whatever else our evil, evil coaches dreamed up.

Once again, I didn't really join the team to compete, but I loved the whole masochism of getting in shape. It felt good to hurt, and to be around a bunch of people who were feeling good and hurting at the same time. It felt good to have an appetite, and to answer it instead of deny it. I could come home after a tough practice and eat gigantic plates of pasta slathered in my mom's homemade hummus. It felt like a new victory. After starving and reaching an acceptable weight, I could return to my old friend—after-school food—and not feel ashamed.

GREEN DAYS

When I arrived at a small liberal arts school tucked away in a lush corner of the Pacific Northwest, I met a gal who had recently gone vegan. She lived on the same floor in the dorm, so we wound up spending a lot of time together. Before I met her, I think I held a lot of the stereotypical views about vegans as people—they're too extreme, for one—and I figured eggs and cheese weren't actual flesh, so the animals weren't really hurt. Those were pretty much the extent of my thoughts on the matter.

My friend was brimming with new-vegan energy and talked my ear off about how great she felt. I might have had a few stars in my eyes (a slight schoolgirl crush, maybe), so I was definitely a captive audience. What can I say? I was seventeen years old, at a college three thousand miles away from where I grew up, a school that didn't give out grades. It was practically a factory for vegans.

College also meant I could eat without anyone watching me, not in the sense that I was used to, anyway. I don't remember what exactly I bought on my first solo trip to the grocery store, but I do remember the bounce in my step. I got to choose my food! I can always find an article somewhere that talks about how unhealthy relationships with food and a negative body image aren't so much about food as they are about control. And I won't disagree.

My new-vegan friend cooked for me, too. Everything tasted fantastic, and it didn't seem hard at all. Changing my diet, cooking for myself, sharing and enjoying meals with other people all helped me see food in a different way, a way that didn't involve shame or rules. I had power over what I ate. I wasn't concerned so much with how the food I was cooking and eating was going to shape my body. In the dark and damp capital of Washington State, my days were looking pretty bright.

One night, the power went out in the dorm, thanks to a windstorm. It was the perfect excuse to stay up late and run wild. On a whim that week at the grocery store, I had decided to buy graham crackers and milk, a kindergarten snack throwback, maybe because I was toying with the age-old grownup/kid dichotomy. Over the course of a long night with no electricity and lots of frolicking through the dark halls, doing things that college kids do, I drank three mugs of milk.

I woke up the next day and felt disgusting. I'm sure many factors were involved, but I blamed the milk. This was right before Thanksgiving and Christmas, so I decided that after navigating the winter holidays at home with the family, I'd go vegan.

The clouds didn't part, angels didn't sing, and no one bestowed a golden halo upon my head. Going vegan wasn't a magic bullet, and it wasn't a panacea for everything that ailed me. I know I still worried about my body and all its imperfections, but, for a while, I didn't blame food or myself—we were all happy together, vegan.

I'll admit it: I was young and dumb, and I said some stupid things when people asked me why I was vegan (the ever-so-common *health or ethics?* question). I was careful when I answered, considered who was asking, and tried hard to make sure I wasn't the preachy vegan. My good answer: *Animals don't need to die for me to live.* My bad answer: *If I wasn't vegan, I'd be, like, five hundred pounds.* From the mouths of babes, indeed.

While I was trying on these new identities at the ripe old age of nearly nineteen, my dad died, unexpectedly. He passed away the day I was riding on a plane to go home for December break. Our relationship was complicated (what father–daughter relationship isn't?). I wasn't even sure I was going to see him during my vacation, and I felt bad and sad and mad about that, which is quite possibly the definition of *complicated*. When I woke up at my mom's house, she was putting a box of tissues in my hand. "Cassandra, I have to tell you something," she said. "Your father died last night."

Since then, I have thought of myself as a sort of continuing study in grief and love and how the push and pull of both shape and change people. The first year after my dad died, I didn't think or care about food or my body at all. Certainly not in that "I must control this to be perfect" way. I was too busy preparing for something else unexpected. Grief scooped my insides out and left me a worried shell.

It was good, in a way, to have my internal gears reset. Obsessing about food and my body holds me back. I know that. I'm grateful in hindsight for the distraction that grief brought. Even though I thought I was such a big girl at college, I knew that losing my dad made me young and green all over again.

WEATHERED DAYS

The first time I bought running sneakers after high-school cross-country and track was when I decided to quit smoking. A few career years of sitting at a desk all day and staring at a computer screen made me feel just antsy enough to do something physically challenging. I was rather fond of smoking and the exciting social realm it involved, but being part of that special little circle wasn't holding the same appeal anymore. Smoking also didn't fit so well with my being vegan, which had an air of health to it, and friends were always surprised. "You smoke?!" was a frequent exclamation. Nobody's perfect, right?

You can't be a smoker and a runner, I told myself, and I made the wise choice. I ran for a little while, but I didn't stick with it. I didn't go back to smoking, though. I remember my knees hurting, and it was always raining (I lived in Seattle at the time). I think those of us who gravitate toward running as a hobby or sport or even profession come from some hearty stock, but I was not quite hearty enough to run in Seattle. My waxy outer layer was not developed, and it felt just plain dumb to voluntarily go out and get rained on.

A few years later, after my first winter in Chicago (which, I might add, included an epic and historic blizzard of three feet of snow in February), I began toying with the idea of running again. I had been working from home for almost a year, and all signs pointed to a need for a change of pace that involved getting out of the house and being active. A lot of women in my online circle of vegan pals ran, and someone mentioned a program called Couch to 5K. I'd been practicing yoga off and on for a while, so I wasn't exactly starting from the couch, but it had been so long since my feet pounded the pavement. The program, which started with easy intervals of walking and running, sounded completely doable.

Within the first week, I knew I was hooked. I had flipped the switch, and I was back to the mindset of being a runner. The streets looked different to me. They were still flat, but they had so much potential. *I* had so much potential. I had muscles in my legs and arms that I hadn't felt in years. These muscles remembered winter track and wall squats. They remembered six-mile runs. It was a great day when my brain caught up to what my body had known all along. My body knew that strength and health—real wellness—are what it needed. Not some self-constructed picture of thinness, and not the terribly small amount of food that it takes. Like those proud days of high school, I had permission to fuel my body again.

LIGHT DAYS

I spend a few hours working and juggling various deadlines, all from the comfortable but small space of my apartment. Sometime around 11:30 A.M., my breakfast has completely worn off, and I reach for a little more fuel. If I can magically clear my desk an hour or so later, I start scrambling around for sweats and sneakers and a little armband that holds my ID and other important cards. If, dare I say, I take a major spill and crack my head open on the sidewalk, then I want the Good Samaritan who finds me to easily locate my insurance information. If it's between thirty-two and eighty degrees outside, I consider myself rather lucky, jam my headphones into my ears, and bust out of the building like I'm being shot out of a cannon.

I start with a few minutes of brisk walking. I smile at the dogs who are out for their own midday constitutional. I breathe a little more deeply and feel very thankful indeed for the three-dimensional world. Aside from the little gadget that will track my time and distance, I feel far away from the electronic world, and that distance feels better than any amount of miles I can physically cover with my feet. I set the timer for twenty minutes, thirty minutes, maybe forty-five minutes, and I just start running. There's an internal shift—it happens every time—when I realize that I've completely let go of what had been preoccupying me before I left. I can't remember it now, as I concentrate on lighter footfalls. I nod at other runners I pass. I wonder how fast I'm going. I start thinking about how great lunch will taste.

When I'm running, I'm testing my body, and I'm trying to make it stronger, not smaller. Strength is what I want, more than rock-hard calves and a flat, flat stomach. I don't want to be the starving waif who has an empty food journal. I want to be healthy and strong. This means I have to eat. Freely. It means I have to eat and run. To cook and feed myself. To tie on my shoes and keep going.

The dark part of me, who still thinks that no one will love the fat latchkey kid, is sometimes the part that gets me out the door and out there to pound the pavement. I'm not all darkness, though, and the more I run, the lighter I feel. I imagine myself during the day as a coil, winding around and around my insides, until I am tight and kinked. When I run, I feel the coil turning in the opposite direction, powering my footsteps and driving the amazing machine of my body as my lungs push my breath in and out. I'm running with every day I've lived before welling up inside of me.

As I stand at the top of the stairs, face flushed, maybe panting a little and stretching out my calves, I know the coil has bloomed open. The remainder of the day is ripe with possibilities. I'm clear again. Full of potential.

7

Fit Fathers, Devoted Dads

Kimatni D. Rawlins

When my two daughters ask me why I decided to go vegan, I think back to dinnertime when I was growing up in the 1970s in Camden, New Jersey. Keeping the fridge and cupboards stocked was problematic for my mother, so my two younger sisters and I would take a vote on what was ideal based on the limited ingredients. Three out of seven days we had "breakfast for dinner," since there was always a carton of eggs, milk, pancake mix, and a few slices of bacon lying around. On special days, we would have BLTs on toasted Wonder Bread—yes, that white bread that turns into paste when wet—layered with mayonnaise and a yokey fried egg. Other nights, my mother would serve fried liver with mashed potatoes or white rice or macaroni.

Over the years, mother worked feverishly on her nursing degree to help my sisters and me escape the immense poverty, minimal education, and debilitating crime of a city that seemed bent on self-destruction. There were no shopping malls, movie theaters, or recreation centers for us kids to escape to. There were, however, bullying, fights, drugs, and free blocks of government cheese that we used to make grilled sandwiches that hardly melted under the heat. Food stamps played an integral role in our food choices and level of nutrition. When times were tough we survived on mayonnaise sandwiches; when times were good we ate out at McDonald's and Roy Rogers. Although Mom made us eat Quaker Oats and corn and peas (the kind that came in frozen bags), our diet mostly consisted of foods that were fried or made with enriched white flour. The only physical activity available to my mother was the dreaded long, weekly walks from the grocery store with heavy bags of sugar, Kool-Aid, and every fattening snack imaginable. She also roller-skated, which burned calories. Yet, we certainly didn't look at any of these activities as exercise, and the foods were what my mother could afford. None of us knew they had the potential to cause heart disease, diabetes, and colon cancer.

I was introduced to a healthier diet by my father. My parents split up shortly after I was born, when they were teenagers. After serving in the Vietnam War, my father found himself in Washington, D.C., where he became a strict vegetarian (vegan by today's standards). When I visited him in the summer and on holidays I inexorably took on this strange pattern of eating. Protein shakes, vitamins the size of grapes, gluten, tofu, soy milk, millet, and fruits and vegetables of all colors, shapes, and flavors replaced the crap I was used to eating. The change was so devastating that I would always break out with rashes when I switched diets. My father said it was the poisons detoxing from my body. Yep, he was officially "mad" in my book. Looking back, he was absolutely right. A former boxer, Pops was lean and muscular and always practiced what he preached.

My father never explained his reasons for becoming a vegetarian and how it led to healthier digestion, growth, and living. He also never showed me how to read labels, and he certainly didn't expound on the nutritional benefits of a meatless and dairy-free diet. My two sisters from my father's side and I would look at each other sideways and just ate the stuff. We also rode bikes, walked to the zoo, swam, went camping, and practiced yoga. My father was fervently in tune with the mind–body connection and even made us meditate.

Each fall, I would return to Camden leaner and stronger than when I left. My mother encouraged me by purchasing a cement weight-set that I employed to work out five days a week. By the age of twelve I was without doubt the strongest kid in the neighborhood. This was useful on the treacherous streets of Camden. Back then we played basketball, football, raced each other on foot, and biked or walked everywhere. Our families didn't have the luxury of modern transportation. Every kid in Camden was fit. More importantly, there were so many bullies looking to pick a fight that speed was a common necessity for escape. I considered myself a peacemaker and saw no moral victory in fighting . . . until later in high school.

High school was a pivotal time for me. My mother moved us out of Camden and into the suburban neighborhood of Voorhees where the education was much better. Soon, I was living out the prototypical story of the kid from the city who goes to school in the 'burbs and makes good. I performed well inside the classroom and out, and gradually developed into one of the top athletes in New Jersey. I won state titles in track and field, excelling in the 100- and 200-yard dash, hurdles, and the long jump. As a 205-pound running back I led my high-school football team to a conference title and a spot in the Group Championship game. I was racking up accolades and awards, as well as recruitment visits from Division One collegiate football programs. It became clear that I would become the first member of my family to attend a Division One university and on a scholarship, no less.

Although I went on to play for North Carolina State and later transferred to the Georgia Institute of Technology, my story soon became one familiar to many college students: heavy drinking began to play a major role in my educational and athletic development. Thinking back, I believe I took in some booze and even an occasional blunt every day of the week. Oftentimes, I went on the field still intoxicated from all-night binges. My focus eroded and my athletic skills diminished. On top of that, the coaches were stuffing us like factory animals. I grew to 225 pounds of pure muscle while chowing down on meat, potatoes, and cheese dishes. Inevitably, I lost my love for the sport and simply showed up in order to graduate.

Afterwards, I started working in various fields in the automotive industry, where my old man had made his career. He published *African Americans on Wheels* automotive magazine, pivotal since his company was the only diverse media outlet in the auto world at the time. Who would have thought, a vegetarian entrepreneur breaking into the upper echelons of big business?

Eventually, I ventured out on my own and founded Automotive

Rhythms Communications, a lifestyle automotive media and marketing portal. This allowed me to travel the globe assessing new automobiles and motorcycles, as well as cuisines that were new to me. Here I was, a kid from Camden, staying in a five-star hotel in Paris and being given the opportunity to try foie gras, frogs' legs, and snails. Unfortunately, with all the traveling and hosted dinners came more eating and drinking to unprecedented levels. By the end of a night, I would typically have consumed nine glasses of wine and a few Johnnie Walker Blacks and sometimes Blues, which typically cost $50 a glass. *How much better could it get?* I thought. This disastrous lifestyle continued for ten more years.

One morning in 2011, I walked into the bathroom, stepped on the scale, and discovered that I weighed more than 250 pounds, but devoid of most of my muscles. Now I was as chubby as a beaver. I looked in the mirror. My face was thick and my skin as dry as a raisin. When I went to the closet, I noticed that I now wore size 42 jeans and 3X shirts. How had this happened? Well, I didn't exactly exercise twice a day like I was back at Ga. Tech, but I still played basketball, flag football, and weightlifted. I had even cut back on the partying and drinking, but my daily diet was only slightly better than what I had grown up with, except that I had given up beef and pork. Nonetheless, chicken cheesesteaks, wings with blue cheese, sugary drinks, chips, and other snacks ran my life. To top it off I was driving everywhere, since Automotive Rhythms always had a fleet of vehicles in the driveway. Why ride a bike when a $100,000 Mercedes-Benz awaited? But enough was enough, and I decided to make a permanent lifestyle change.

The very next day, I signed up for the Men's Health Urbanathlon, a nine to eleven–mile run through the streets of Chicago, New York, and San Francisco. Training for the event required four days of running activities, alternating between distance and sprints, and two days of strength training. I decided to run the Chicago race first because I wanted the chance to climb the hundreds of stadium steps at Soldier Field—where my hero, the running back Walter Payton, played—as part of the course. By the time race day came around five months later, I had lost twenty-five pounds, toned up quite a bit, and stopped drinking alcohol completely. Additionally, I progressed from not being able to run a mere mile without breathing heavily to checking off eight, ten, and twelve miles minus the hesitation or strain. Best of all, I had dropped four waist and two shirt sizes. It felt good to be trim again.

Since most of what I had been by taught by public educational institutions regarding food was wrong, I set out to educate myself by reading a book a week, watching documentaries such as *Forks over Knives*, and attending seminars and health conferences. Slowly, light was being shed on the childhood eating habits I had learned from my father. Once I understood that we must eat whole foods from the earth to meet the balance of vitamins, minerals, and phytonutrients our bodies need, I went on a mission to rid myself of all meat, dairy, and processed foods. My next challenge was a full marathon while operating on vegan fuel. Once I completed that task I knew I would never turn back. More importantly, I've gotten down to my high school weight of 202 pounds, can still bench my max of 405 pounds when I train for four months, and regained my sprinting capabilities, which helps me run a 21-minute 5K at age 40.

But it wasn't enough that I was getting healthier; I needed my wife and daughters, ages nine and six at the time, to be healthy too. I began to make subtle changes, replacing fattening snacks with celery and hummus, sodas with fresh kale and pineapple juice or a strawberry smoothie made with coconut milk. Dinnertime now involved whole grains such as brown rice, millet, and quinoa, and cruciferous veggies like spinach, broccoli, and collard greens. With sadness, I realized how costly the healthier organic path to eating could be, and understood why my mother couldn't nourish us as she wanted to. Maybe if the U.S. government subsidized produce like they do meat and dairy we would live in a healthier country. My wife and I also began involving the kids in as much physical activity as possible, including swim class, soccer, dance, and family bike riding. Now my six-year-old likes to hit the punching bag with me.

Even that wasn't enough. I looked around me and saw all the fast food, sugary snacks, and excessive Internet and television use that have supplanted home-cooked meals and active living to a point where obesity and lethargy are accepted as the norm. For that reason, I founded Fit Fathers, an inspirational and life enhancing movement to help families focus on their well-being and that of their children. The program offers fitness workouts and routines, recipes for wholesome meals, nutritional food shopping advice, childhood activity integrations for busy parents, recommendations on degenerative-disease prevention and fitness-friendly places to travel, and of course encouragement to keep mothers and fathers on top of their game. Now I am a certified fitness trainer as well as certified in plant-based nutrition from T. Colin Campbell's eCornell.com program.

So when my daughters ask me why I and our family decided to go vegan, I tell them that it is the best food in the world and that our bodies need nourishment from foods that grow from trees, roots, and plants rather than foods that are born. We love animals and they deserve to be free, just as we humans do. Over the years, I have learned to distinguish between eating as an omnivore and as a herbivore, and ultimately chose the better path. But I have no regrets with the manner in which I was raised. It has shaped me into the person I am today and allows me to engage with those who currently live the life I used to. The journey towards health and happiness is waiting for us; sometimes we just need a little encouragement from those who have run the same path and completed the journey.

8

A Well-Rounded Vegan

JL Fields

I started running the year I turned thirty-nine. I had just made goal on yet another diet. But this time, after fifteen years of on-and-off-again smoking, I was ready to quit that, too. Fearful I would regain the weight I started running. Reluctantly. I hated it.

I didn't run just a little bit. My first race was a 10K; why run 3.1 miles when I could run 6.2? A few months later, I ran a half-marathon and said to my runner husband, "I'll never run a full marathon." He laughed. A year later, I ran a full marathon. Six months after that, I ran another one. After that second marathon I said, "I'll never run a marathon again." He didn't laugh and, so far, I haven't. But I did run seventeen half-marathons in a five-year timespan and have competed in over ten triathlons.

All to stay skinny.

Here's the kicker—I still had to diet while doing all of that running. Counting carbs while training for a marathon. Cuckoo, I tell you.

Here's what a calendar year of running looked like:

January: *Uh, oh, holiday pounds!*
February–March: *Diet and build up to a big race*
April–August: *Race (race, race) and oh-so-skinny*
September–December: *Less racing, more eating*
January: *Uh, oh. Rounder.*

Every. Single. Year.

I was vegetarian during this time. In fact, I turned vegetarian just a few years before I took up running. I was in a small village in the Rift Valley in Kenya for an auspicious occasion—the nonprofit organization where I served as executive director was opening a safe house for girls fleeing female genital mutilation—and my colleagues and I were the guests of honor. Early in the day, an elder from the community brought a goat to the site of the celebration as a sign of his support of our effort. There were whispers among the female community leaders at the event; one woman leaned over and said, "It's like he's giving away a Mercedes-Benz." The goat was marched past us and disappeared with the elder behind a building. I can't even remember what the goat looked like as, feeling uncomfortable, I averted my eyes. It did not take long for us to understand that the goat was going to be slaughtered. That evening, we were offered the goat for dinner. I told myself that to refuse it would be an affront to our hosts. Essentially, I felt as if I met a goat and then I ate him. It was at that moment that I understand the implications of what I ate. There was a cost associated—a life.

I became a vegetarian the next day.

Back in the States, I found a number of vegetarian options in popular diet plans such as the South Beach Diet and Weight Watchers, and they worked. I would get skinny by spring and run like hell during the summer to keep the weight off.

Three years ago, I was ready for another January diet. Which one this time? I opted for a nutritional cleanse with a yoga instructor; it seemed so much gentler. For sixteen days I abstained from wheat, sugar, caffeine, alcohol—and dairy. At the end of the cleanse I realized I had eaten only one animal product during the entire time—a single hard-boiled egg. I was an egg away from being vegan!

So I went vegan. Without one thought about animals. But I had found a new way to lose weight.

I kept running and doing marathons for another year. And guess what happened at the end of that year? Yep, it was time to go on a diet. The miraculous vegan diet didn't make me skinny. I was a round vegan. I sat down with my nutritionist to talk about my January plan and she said something deeply profound and, frankly, life-changing.

She asked a very simple question: "But what if this is your weight? Have you considered buying bigger clothes?"

Holy shit! No, actually I had not considered either as viable options.

I went shopping the next day. I bought a pair of jeans, a dress, and a skirt. All in my December weight. I went to work the following week in my new dress and was greeted with "Did you lose weight?"

I replied with a simple, "No." I had just spent the first four years of my forties chasing the weight of my twenties. I was chasing skinny. I stopped. I decided to embrace my rounder body.

When I shifted away from the desire to be thin, I was able to connect to my veganism in a completely different and unexpected way. In my bigger jeans, I visited Woodstock Farm Animal Sanctuary in upstate New York and fell in love with a goat named Clover. I began to make regular visits to the sanctuary where I would pet and play with her, as well as many other furry and feathered creatures on the farm. Clover had been saved from slaughter in Yonkers and was living a full, round-bellied life. A completely opposite life from that of the goat I met in Africa.

I went vegetarian because of a goat; I went vegan because of health and diet; and in that moment, with a rescued goat, I set another goal. I would remain vegan for animals. When I stopped focusing on my size and how I looked, my heart grew bigger, my spirit rounder. My focus on others—people, animals—helped me grow inside as I adjusted to growing outside.

I resumed my running schedule. I had registered for a race but I lacked the motivation to train. It was the first time that I was training for races in which the motivation was not related to my weight. And I didn't want to do it! I offered all kinds of excuses. In the meantime, I was doing something extraordinary. I wasn't dieting. I was eating bread. I was creating vegan recipes. I wasn't depriving myself. In fact, it was quite the opposite. I began eating a healthful, well-balanced diet that included vegetables, fruit, legumes, grains, and nuts and seeds. I didn't count food to be less—in grams and calories; rather, I counted food to be *more*—five to seven servings of vegetables, three or more servings of grains, three or more servings of beans. I was more healthy and stayed full. I laughed when people suggested I was depriving myself on a vegan diet. *Are you kidding?* I thought. *I have never enjoyed a more diverse diet. Kale, quinoa, and tempeh—oh my!*

From my new vantage point of living a balanced life and eating a balanced, filling diet, my relationship with running became complicated. In my mind's eye, it became the new punisher. Whereas bagels were last year's devil, the empowered, rounder me pointed my finger at running as the oppressor. I didn't race that April half-marathon. I did eke out a triathlon later in the summer, ending my season injured because I hadn't trained properly. I didn't run for another six months.

A year later, I found myself in a place of what felt like overall balance. I had grown accustomed to my new weight and size. Not only was my body fuller, but my life—from diet to work to love—felt truly well-rounded. And I was desperate to start running again, after being sidelined with an injury for so many months. But resuming my running was like dating a new partner. It was no longer familiar to me. I didn't run as fast as I had when I was skinny. I wasn't targeting a race, so I didn't have a goal or purpose. I realized I was running because I missed it, and because I loved it. I had become that runner on the street with the stupid grin. I was just so happy to be able to move my body in a familiar way, minus the punishment.

I'm not a skinny vegan. I don't live the hype many are promised before they eat a plant-based diet. I am that round vegan that makes some "health vegans" cringe. I am that vegan who now connects more to the ethics of the word "vegan" than to the health benefits and, while on a journey of compassion toward animals, became kinder to herself. I am the round vegan who unapologetically shows up at running races and triathlons wearing a "No Meat Athlete" tech shirt, knowing full well people may be scratching their heads wondering why she's not a waif.

My vegan running isn't about getting smaller. It's about being bigger and bolder. Joyfully rounder—in body and in spirit.

9

A Magic and Peaceable Kingdom

Gordon E. Harvey

My two boys woke with a fever and those burning, red eyes that signify only one thing: the flu. Their mother and I panicked. We were just days away from a scheduled family vacation to Disney World, and I could see money, time, and effort all being washed down the drain. We bathed in hand sanitizer, sprayed disinfectant on anything that moved—including the kids—and washed our hands with the fervor of religious zealots. We took every precaution imaginable. In spite of this, I woke up the morning after the kids' fever broke, feeling the symptoms myself. I knew I had caught the flu.

I rushed to the clinic, desperate for some miracle drug that would allow me to travel to see Mickey Mouse. I knew something was wrong when four different nurses took my vitals. The physician broke the news: "Gordon, you don't have the flu. You have dangerously high blood pressure. We're going to give you this pill, have you lie in a dark room for a while, and if your blood pressure doesn't come down a bit, we're going to send you to the emergency room."

I'm no medical professional, but I am fairly certain that if you want someone to relax so his blood pressure can fall, this is not the best way to do it. Nevertheless, there I lay in a darkened room, watching my life flash before my eyes and thinking, *Is this the end? Am I dying? What about my sons?! I need to see them grow up and become men! I'm their dad, not a human time bomb in a dark medical examination room! What the hell have I done to myself?*

My blood pressure reduced just enough for me to be allowed to go home. The physician put me on blood-pressure medication, told me to stop eating salt, and ordered me to start losing weight. I was allowed to travel, so the trip to Disney World took place after all, but it was the strangest of dichotomies—wondering how much longer I had to live while walking around the "happiest place on Earth." It would have been nice to use some Disney magic to remove all this fat from my body. I walked a great deal, eschewed fried foods, and noticed all the other obese people in the park. I didn't want to be one of those people anymore. I wanted to change, to be fit, to live a healthy life.

This is what I had done, or rather, eaten: fresh, hand-patted burgers every Saturday night, fried chicken every Sunday lunch, some form of beef on every other night of the week. Butter, milk, cheese, fat, sugar—all staples in my childhood diet. You have to understand, I am a child of the American South. Butter and lard, and lots of it, finds its way in every dish. Want some green beans? You won't get them without huge chunks of bacon or ham. Vegetables? Sure. I loved them, as long as they were baked potatoes, fried potatoes, or mashed potatoes.

Don't blame my parents, or theirs either. This was a cultural thing. It was all they knew. My mom quit school in tenth grade to support her dirt-poor Alabama family. A disabled brother, a blind mother, and a coal-miner father who died long before I was born left her with no choice but to work. She grew up in poverty and made a promise to herself that her children would never know want. My dad fared better. The son of a master machinist, he traveled to South and Central America working for Standard Oil and later the U.S. Atomic Energy Commission in Oak Ridge, Tennessee. They blessed me with all I've ever needed to grow up happy and well-adjusted. And they taught me gratitude: never to take for granted what I have and to know that hard work—as exhibited in their lives—is more important than anything.

Nonetheless, forty years of bad eating had taken a toll on my body. I had tried and cheated on many diets, but had eventually quit on all of them. After returning from Disney World, I decided to start running. Oh, I had run some in college, and in high school I played football and wrestled. But it was something I did as support for other athletic endeavors, or as punishment. I was currently active, mind you, but primarily through yoga, spinning classes, officiating soccer, and some step aerobics. I decided that running would be the solution for me—my magic wand, so to speak.

The first time I ran, I had trouble breathing. One mile felt like forever. But the strangest thing happened. After the run, I felt *alive*. In following runs, I reminded myself that every stride was prolonging my life and helping me lose weight. I registered for three 5Ks in three months. I couldn't get enough of that feeling of accomplishment at the finish line of a race. I never thought I'd run anything longer than a 5K, though. My brother-in-law, then training for the Los Angeles Marathon, once asked me if I'd ever consider running 26.2 miles. I laughed at the question. "No way," I said. "I'm a short-distance man. Marathons are crazy!"

Three months later, I approached a colleague about training me for the Disney Marathon. I had realized that I needed a bigger goal. Two of my earlier trips to Disney World had taken place during Marathon Weekend, when runners get to race through all four parks as visitors cheer them on. I got goosebumps just watching them. It made perfect sense to run my first marathon in a place that had brought my family great joy. I set the January 2009 Disney Marathon as my goal and spent the next few months "Running to Disney," which was also the name of a blog and podcast I produced to document my training. Every long run became a milestone in my life (and an excuse to eat unhealthful stuff as a reward), and every week brought me closer to one of the greatest days of my life.

They say that the feelings associated with your first marathon, like your first kiss, can never be replicated. So, with that in mind I snapped pictures, recorded video and audio, and tried to take in every sensation. It was a long, hard race on a hot, sunny day. I didn't run it fast (6:10), but I ran it proudly. As I approached the finish line and heard the announcer call my name, tears streamed down my face. I had done it. I had done something unheard of for a guy like me. I scanned the crowd and, across the chain-link fence separating the spectators from the racers, saw my kids, who were wearing T-shirts that said "My Dad Ran the Disney Marathon."

Sobbing from relief, exhilaration, and exhaustion, I told them I loved them.

Crossing that finish line was a magical moment for me. I floated for two months. I wore my marathon hat and shirt everywhere. I sipped coffee from the marathon mug. And I kept eating a lot. Something was missing from the equation. The early weight loss when I first started running had fallen off. I had even regained a little weight. I was five-foot-nine inches tall and weighed 239 pounds—not the body weight most conducive to running growth.

So, with a new marathon goal and a new eating plan in place, I began the fall with a renewed purpose. Enter Megan, a friend whom I had met through social media, who offered to assist me with nutritional improvement and my running. Her compassionate veganism taught me a lot about making good food choices. By the turn of 2010, I had become a vegetarian, a fairly easy transition. After researching vegan substitutes and ingredients and label reading, I went vegan that March. Over a few months, I had gone from a carnivore of the highest level to a vegan, with compassion for my own body, the environment, and my fellow earthlings.

I now weigh 156 lbs and have lost seventy-five pounds since July 2009; and ninety-two pounds since early 2007 when this running odyssey began. Over the past four years I've eaten more fruits and veggies than I did in my first forty-two years of life. My cholesterol has dropped; I have more energy; I'm wearing clothing sizes even the junior high–school me wouldn't have considered wearing. And that blood pressure medication that I was told I'd have to take for the rest of my life? My doctor took me off it and said I was a role model for my new lifestyle.

It has taken a while for me to wrap my head around what has happened to my mind, my body, and my outlook on life. As an endurance athlete I have found that the vegan lifestyle not only assists in weight loss and cardiovascular health, it also has fostered fast recovery from hard workouts and quickened endurance growth. I've gone from a 6:10 marathon time in January 2009 to a 3:28 in February 2011. I feel more alive, more joyful, more self-aware than at any time in my life. I feel, well, cleaner.

While I became vegan through the health door, I have since embraced its concern for the environment and compassion to animals. I've experienced remarkable encounters with horses, cows, sheep, dogs, and even squirrels that left a profound mark on me. Realizing that I am but a small part of a larger world of living creatures is moving me in ways I never expected. Last spring, during long training bicycle rides, I stopped to snap pictures of farm animals. I stood by the fence, and a horse came up to me and let me pet her nose. She looked at me with deep brown eyes and I felt touched in a way I've never known. I experienced a sort of kinship, two beings sharing a moment of discovery and enlightenment.

The next weekend, I stopped to snap a picture of a cow. But as I stood by the fence, six other cows came up to the fence alongside the first one. They looked at me. I looked at them. We just stared at each other. I kept thinking: *What's going on here, with these animals and me?* Were they thinking: *Hey, let's go look at the funny human?* Or was there a deeper connection between us? Could they sense I was harmless? Did they know who and what I had become? I like to think it is the latter. That we *are* connected. That we all deserve a chance to live our own lives, whether animal or human.

I've never felt this before in my life. It's similar to the thoughts I have about my kids. The emotional response I get when I see them just being themselves: loving, goofy, happy, sad—even arguing and fighting. As the only vegan in my family, it's not always easy to juggle my new lifestyle with my role as a parent. I want my boys to make their own choices in life, but I strive to model vegan compassion for them. I try to point out how their love for our dog Rookie should also be given to other animals that society has labeled "filthy" or "edible," such as cows and pigs. I know that one day these seeds I'm planting will grow, and I must be patient and let my kids have their own moments of self-discovery and self-actualization.

Running opened the door for all of this. It led me to veganism. It led me to new friends. It led me to greater health. And in turn, veganism has opened the door to my becoming a better runner, an endurance athlete with a fitness level that I could never have imagined. My body is healthy. My heart is happy. My soul is fulfilled. I am connected to my world in a deeper, more profound way. And I love it all.

10

For the Love of Lentils

Christine Frietchen

"You, who dare insult lentil soup, sweetest of delicacies."

—ARISTOPHANES

They're tiny little things, aren't they? I think they look like flying saucers. I like to pour them through my hands, feeling them rush between my fingers, not so much like sand, but like smooth river stones. If you pour them in a bowl and plunge your hands in, they feel wonderful. Sure, lentils are better to eat than play with, but the sound of dry lentils being poured into a bowl is serenely soothing.

We're making up for lost time, lentils and I. We only met a few short years ago, and our age difference is stark: Lentils have been around for at least 9,500 years—lentil seeds have been found in archeological digs in the Middle East and are one of the world's oldest cultivated plants. They're mentioned in the Bible several times. In Genesis 25:29–34, Esau gives away his birthright to his twin brother Jacob in exchange for lentils and bread. By most interpretations, this was seen as a rotten trade, but I'm not so sure; lentils and a chunk of bread are pretty darn good.

The earliest recipe for lentils might have come from Anthimus, a sixth-century Byzantine physician who advocated food as medicine in his book *On the Observance of Food*. He recommends slow-cooking the lentils, then adding a little vinegar, ground sumac, and salt, along with olive oil and whole coriander seeds. The recipe still works today, and it is seriously good. (You can find sumac in a Middle-Eastern grocery store; zaatar, a spice blend that includes sumac, is also delicious.)

Lentils have only existed in my world for about fifteen years. I remember my first encounter with them, in an Indian restaurant called Haveli in New York City's East Village (it's still there). I tried mulligatawny there for the first time—a heavenly creamy soup with curry and vegetables. Back then, I wasn't yet vegan, and I wasn't yet a runner, but I remember that first taste of lentils—the little "pop" of each perfectly cooked legume. It was a few years later, after my life and health changed immeasurably, that lentils reasserted themselves as the perfect running food.

I was not the sporty child. I was far more interested in the books arranged in the Leavenworth, Kansas, public library. My first crush when I was thirteen wasn't on the class clown or soccer kid; it was on the town librarian's son. The smell of old paper was far more exciting to me than the smell of a ball glove. I nonetheless put up a front, playing lackluster softball through a couple years of high school, shifting my weight from side to side in the outfield, waiting for the inning to be over, counting the minutes until I could bury my nose in *Little Women* or *Pride and Prejudice*.

College was a joy; no one cared if you were athletic. Smart was now cool. Irony and sarcasm were hip. I piled on the books, almost as quickly as I packed on the pounds. My Midwestern meat-and-potatoes education ill prepared me for living on my own. I relied on Hamburger Helper, pots of chili, and a lot of macaroni and cheese. I don't ever recall taking a nutrition class in high school. My idea of buying healthful food was choosing the lean ground beef. Fast food was cheap and easy. It's fair to say that even while I obsessed over my growing weight, I thought not one iota about food other than choosing that night's pizza toppings or which variety of packaged noodle mix to make.

Ten years later, I'm living in the home of the New York City Marathon, and a friend is running in it. I'd worked with Lee for a few years, and I was jealous. She was fit, strong, and confident. She prioritized her health and made time for running while the rest of us worked late into the night to finish projects. She pissed off pretty much everyone by ditching us to hit the track. I'd never met anyone like that, and I was aghast. I'd tried to lose weight for years at that point, never getting very far, and had settled into my societal role as the fat bridesmaid in all the weddings; the funny, outgoing friend who is never a threat to anyone.

But when Lee challenged me to start running—she volunteered to join me in a five-mile race later in the year—I was flattered into buying my first pair of running shoes (New Balance!). The next year, I won a lottery entry into the New York City Marathon.

I ran that first marathon fueled on a conventional diet—all the stuff the running books said I was supposed to eat: pasta, yogurt, lean meat, and eggs. I faithfully followed the training plans in marathon books. I built up my mileage little by little over four months. And I admit, I had an agenda beyond completing the race: I thought I'd surely drop a few pounds running so many training miles. I figured that running twenty-, thirty-, and forty-mile weeks would turn me into the slim, fit person I desperately wanted to be. In those four months of training, I lost a grand total of four pounds.

I finished the 26.2 miles in 5:06, respectable for a first marathon but hardly remarkable. And for the last five miles, I was miserable, barely keeping my feet moving in what I call a survival shuffle. After resting for a couple of weeks, I told myself I should start doing some short runs again, but my heart wasn't in it. I just stopped running. For eight years.

Around the time I bought my first bag of dried lentils, I started to really get back into running.

Following that first marathon, I'd been flirting slowly with vegetarianism, then veganism, in a way that probably sounds familiar to lots of people: I was dating a vegetarian, and I stopped buying meat. I found I didn't miss it: didn't miss the coppery smell, the pool of blood on the bottom of the little Styrofoam packages, the slimy feel on my fingers.

And once the meat was gone, a whole new vegetable world revealed itself. New York City's farmers' markets had types of squash I'd never seen. I'd only ever met pumpkins growing up, and those were turned into Halloween art projects, not dinner. I met ten kinds of peppers. I'd only been to first base with bell peppers in Kansas, and even then, only as the ornamental filling for fajitas, next to the fatty strips of steak and dry chicken. I met a dozen types of lettuce beyond the nutritionally void "iceberg." I tasted my way through twenty varieties of apple, a world away from the rock-hard Red Delicious apples that served as the token school-lunchroom fruit.

During those years of nascent vegetarianism, I wouldn't say I cooked so much as "assembled." My boyfriend and I made myriad salads, pots of veggie chili, piles of black beans with guacamole. But I was still clinging to cheese, the last vestige of that old heartland upbringing. It took a screening of the documentary *Forks over Knives* to nudge me over the edge into full-on vegan. I loved it.

Ditching cheese made me feel amazing. My heartburn went away; I had more energy, I just felt . . . *clean*. And I started running. And swimming, and biking. This was a full-on honeymoon; I felt joy when I ran in a way I never did while training for that first marathon. I hummed bad '80s songs in my head as I ran loops around Brooklyn's Prospect Park. I pushed off my toes with a springy zeal. I made new running friends, with whom I talked breathlessly about minimalist running, compression gear, and race nutrition.

I was having so much fun that I hardly noticed I was getting faster. I started entering races again. In the first race I'd entered in eight years—a 10-mile race in Prospect Park—I found I'd improved on my per-minute time by more than two minutes. I finished eleventh in my age group; I'd never finished under 150th before. And this from the non-athletic, non-competitive Kansas kid!

I began to relish racing—pushing myself to the front near the starting line rather than hanging out in the back with the walkers. I spotted runners ahead of me, trained my focus on picking them off, and raced with people who had no idea I had them in my crosshairs. I started to fancy myself an athlete. I began thinking about trying another marathon.

And I started thinking about lentils again. With my weekly mileage edging up, I was constantly hungry. I knew I needed a longer-lasting energy source if I was going to put in the fifty-mile weeks that go along with serious marathon training. At a local Middle Eastern café, I thought, *This tabouleh would be pretty great if I threw some lentils in it.* I started experimenting at home.

My first few clumsy dates with lentils didn't go so well. The first batch I overcooked into a mushy, bitter mess. The next batch suffered the opposite fate: I used too much water, but still managed to undercook them. The third batch? Hallelujah! One cup of dry lentils, two cups of water, a pinch of salt. Bring to a boil, then turn down the heat and simmer for twenty minutes. Water magically absorbs, plumping each little flying saucer without compromising the toothy outer shell. Little lenses pop satisfyingly in your mouth. And a realization: Now I'm cooking stuff, really cooking.

Turns out, lentils are a fabulous running food. Their soluble fiber provides slow-burn energy while their insoluble fiber keeps you regular—very helpful for pre-race mornings. Lentils have the third-highest fiber content among legumes, nuts, and seeds—behind only soy and hemp. Meat eaters are forever telling vegans (especially female vegans) that we can't possibly be getting enough iron, but lentils are loaded with it. Iron is a component of hemoglobin, which helps get oxygen from your lungs to the rest of your cells, providing energy and stamina to the whole body. Perfect for runners.

My first successful experiment was a pimped-up version of tabouleh, inspired by that moment in the Middle Eastern restaurant. I combined lentils with bulgur, veggies, handfuls of parsley, mint, and dill. I added loads of garlic and lemon juice, plus a drizzle of olive oil. I could make a big batch of it in the morning or at night, stick it in the fridge, and the flavors would all mellow out and get cozy with one another. Then it was there after my run, when I needed protein to aid recovery. But it was also terrific pre-run: the bulgur provided whole-grain carbs; the lemon, herbs, and garlic added a huge kick of mouth-puckering goodness.

I felt so well that I chose my second marathon: I'd be racing a spring marathon in New Jersey, nine years after my first attempt. All through the previous late summer and fall, I swam, biked, and ran. And I ate those lentils and that tabouleh salad. Lentils fill you up, but a cup of cooked lentils has just 230 calories. The bathroom scale finally began to budge. Without meat and dairy weighing me down, and with clean whole foods going in—foods I cooked myself—I felt I could push myself longer and harder than I'd ever imagined as a lazy teenager. Running became easy, and I looked forward to dropping into my "zone" at around mile three—that ecstatic moment where your feet find their cadence, your breath regulates, your shoulders relax, and your mind starts humming to your heart's beat.

And that's the addiction. The endorphins kick in; moving either foot stops feeling like an individual effort and starts feeling like an effortless glide. I begin to feel the tiny moment in my stride where I'm actually suspended in air before the next footfall.

Then comes the Zen. My mind starts to float dreamily, like those surreal moments just before you fall asleep when you're neither fully awake but not quite dreaming. Anything seems possible. Maybe this time I'll find myself sprinting through the treetops, running over the surface of the lake, bounding over boulders. And it's not that I'm a fast runner—but in those moments of suspended animation, I'm a gazelle.

During my winter training runs, I became a gazelle in the snow. Winter running is a special thing. No fair-weather runner, you. You're the die-hard. Your family (my family) starts calling you crazy. And the more extreme the temps, the more fun to brag: a twenty-mile training run in fifteen degrees? Yeah, that's just a normal Saturday. Half-marathon in the sleet, trail running in powdery snow? All of it just makes your runs more interesting, spontaneous, and extra beautiful.

Crazy is its own brand of joyful abandon. The number of fellow runners on the road drops to almost nothing, and you find yourself part of a cold-weather brotherhood. I find myself nodding to other runners, a tip of the hat to our obsessive hobby. It's better if you don't know the temperature out there. Just pile on the layers and go. Don't think too much.

Lentils again are your friend! Everybody has a recipe for lentil soup, but I make mine with chunks of winter squash, onion, carrot, and celery. Apple and curry give it a luscious sweetness, and cayenne helps clear your winter sinuses. It's the perfect comfort food in the darkness of winter while you bide your time for the season to change to spring, when all of the hibernating "seasonal" runners emerge from their cold-weather hideaways to crowd the trails and running paths once more.

Lentils have a traditional role in the seasons of life, too. In traditional Jewish mourning, spherical foods, including bagels, eggs, and lentils, are eaten as part of a meal of condolence to symbolize the circular cycle of life and death. This is the first meal that mourners are expected to eat after the death of a loved one. And in other cultures, lentils also have a role at the beginning of life; in Ethiopia, soft lentils are the first solid food given to babies. It makes sense: they are so easy on the stomach.

I completed my second marathon—my first vegan, lentil-fueled marathon—in 3:58:46, more than an hour faster than my first attempt nine years prior. Later that year, I knocked out second- and third-place sprint triathlon age-group titles. I completed an Olympic triathlon and a half Ironman. I'm only getting started. By my next marathon, I'd knocked a further five minutes off my time. I'm going to keep running as long as my legs, and my lentils, will let me.

In the original Grimm version of "Cinderella," Cindy's stepmother challenges her to pick lentils out of a pile of ash. If she's successful, she can go to the ball. Cinderella manages the task, but her stepmother refuses to let her go anyway. Of course, Cinderella soon goes from lentil-collecting ash girl to the belle of the ball. And that's how lentils and running make me feel: beautiful, important, powerful, unstoppable. And also like Cinderella, fiercely competitive. Cindy got the prince in the end. As for me? I'll take the lentils.

WINTER RUNNER'S SOUP
CURRIED LENTILS WITH SQUASH

It takes extra motivation to run in winter, particularly when the temperatures dip below freezing and you're running in snow. But it's also quiet and beautiful, and there's a special freedom in being out in the arctic chill. This hearty soup is speedy to make, and quick to warm you when you get home from ten miles in the frozen tundra.

SERVES: 6
PREP TIME: 20 minutes
COOKING TIME: 20 minutes

1 large onion
1 large clove garlic, minced
1 medium carrot, chopped
1 celery stalk, chopped
1 Tbsp. curry powder
¼ Tsp. cayenne (or to taste)
6–7 cups vegetable stock or broth
4 cups butternut squash, peeled and chopped
1 cup dry lentils
1 large apple, peeled, cored, and chopped
Juice of 1 lemon
1 bay leaf

In a large stock pot, sauté the onion and garlic until tender. Add the carrot and celery and sauté for two or three minutes. Add the curry and cayenne, stirring to coat. Add the vegetable stock, squash, lentils, apple, lemon, and bay leaf. Bring to a boil; turn down heat and simmer until vegetables and lentils are tender, about 20 minutes, and remove bay leaf. You can purée about half of the soup if you like. Season with salt and pepper. That's it.

THINKING

11

Ruminations of a Vegan Non-Runner (Who Runs)

Jasmin Singer

I am not a runner.

I once heard an interview with someone who had recently completed a marathon—not her first one, mind you—and she said the same thing. She was not a runner either; that is not how she thought of herself. She was a mother, a nurse, a Jersey girl. Runners were other people, the ones who wore sweat-wicking clothing bearing lists of their sponsors. They got in thirty-plus miles on Sundays, peed on trails without hesitation, and had Second Skin in their glove compartment at all times. They spoke their own language, full of phrases like "runner's trots" and "black toenails." They didn't drink on Saturday nights. They said things like "Tomorrow I do hills," as if it were a new recreational drug. Runners were a specific breed.

This feeling of being separate from those who call themselves "runners" is one I keenly relate to. I am a New Yorker, a pit-bull mom, a lesbian. I'm a partner, a craftster, a writer. I am an activist. I am a vegan. A runner, though?

I am not a runner.

It is 1991. I am that fat kid in the back of gym class. I am made fun of to the likes of a *20/20* special on bullying. I am not a happy kid in the real world, so I never hesitate to jump head first into my preferred world of make-believe. Soon I make make-believe real by becoming an actress, the one who always gets the role of the quirky best friend, the comic relief, the one with the good number in Act II. I am going to be famous for my timing. Next, I am that teenager who smokes weed and makes overly dramatic statements that worry some and cause others to roll their eyes. I wear heavy eyeliner and listen to Patti LuPone mix-tapes. I move on. I am a broke twenty-something who writes terrible poetry and regularly eats a huge bag of potato chips in one sitting. I get big crushes on inappropriate people. I am in therapy for many years, and, much to the discomfort of near-strangers, talk about it readily. I like to believe I am searching for something.

In my late twenties, I actually find it. I hone in on what I am good at and I get a job with an animal rights organization, adding deep meaning to my un- (or perhaps self-) focused life. I discover true love, and grasp onto it for dear life. I become a dog person. I move my insecurities out of the door and move my home to lower Manhattan. I move my schedule around to encompass activism and writing and I move my heart to my unlikely, yet deeply beautiful relationship with a woman who is a generation older than I. But I do not move my legs.

My thirties start with a mental explosion. I find out from my doctor that I am on my way to heart disease, despite my long-time veganism. I am—*oh my God how did I manage to ignore that this was happening?*—a hundred pounds overweight. Somewhere in between leading protests and writing articles, enjoying life and discovering love, I have lost sight of my physical well-being. My sky-high triglycerides slap me in the face and I find myself confronting physical problems much more common for people twice my age. I become someone who juices, who eats water-sautéed stir-fries, who has desserts made of carob and dates. I become the source of raised eyebrows and quiet conversations. I am sought out by those who struggle with their health, their mood, their weight.

I juice cleanse, repeatedly. In the first year, I lose seventy-five pounds. In the second, I lose the remaining twenty-five. I am what they call a success story.

But I am still not a runner.

Even after I made the uncharacteristic decision to take up the extremely foreign (to me) sport of running, one of the reasons I continued to struggle with defining myself as a runner—aside from my personal history of feigning cramps to get out of gym class—is that running, unlike activism, just doesn't seem important enough to me. Activism is at the core of my self-identity. It is outwardly directed; it demands constant effort and attention. Running, for me, is just something I do. While it has managed to become a huge part of my life—the subject of seemingly unending conversations, Google searches, and (second-hand) shopping expeditions— it is intimate, private, and grows out of a desire to achieve personal goals. Nevertheless, I've learned that running does have its place in my role as an animal rights activist and steadfast advocate of veganism. As I have come to understand, it is in many ways essential not only to my energy and focus, but also to my faith in the possibility of change.

I don't know why I picked up my running shoes for the first time, at age thirty-one. It's not like I ever had any inclination toward athleticism in my life. My propensity always went in the opposite direction. I preferred sitting to standing, escalators to stairs, valet parking to searching for a spot. At airports, I would always take the electronic, Jetsons-esque path, even if I had no luggage. Though I knew exercise was good for you, still, somehow, my busy schedule allowed me to pretend that I just didn't have the time. A moment of exercise was, I felt, a moment I would never again get back, a moment I just couldn't spare. As an animal rights activist, I easily rationalized my decision: If I spent time exercising, I would be taking away time from saving animals. How could anyone argue with such altruism?

But then a few things began to push me toward movement of the physical kind. First, when I started to lose weight, my energy level became otherworldly, almost frenetic. Also, because of my frequent juice-fasting, I became concerned with my metabolism slowing down. In truth, another reason was plain vanity. With such a drastic weight loss sometimes comes stubborn loose skin with a mind of its own. It can be an unsightly and annoying side effect of getting your health in order. Somewhere in my head I figured that the only way to handle this skin, this energy, this plodding metabolism, was to get up and go. So I got up and went.

Immediately—as in, within two blocks—my left knee started throbbing and my side was stitched with cramps. The yoga clothes

I had found at the bottom of my drawer (from an ill-fated moment of "om") were too big, so as I jog-limped on the Hudson River walkway, I was literally holding up my pants. My ratty old sneakers had no cushioning, so my feet ached. I made it a mile out and turned right around, ready to make the trek back home where I would reward myself with a hearty smoothie and a cup of unsweetened cocoa—my newest pleasures in life, replacing chips and peanut-butter bomb cake.

But right before I turned around, as I paused to catch my breath, I accidentally took in the view from where I stood in Lower Manhattan. Had I any breath left in my lungs, it would have been taken away right at that moment, by that exquisite, impeccable sight. In front of me was the Statue of Liberty, standing tall in the midst of the dark, glistening river. On my right was the skyline, beginning with buildings so close I could literally touch them if I took just ten steps, and stretching all the way up to Midtown, the Theatre District, which even from thirty blocks away, was still electric with art, noise, expression—all the reasons I moved to New York in the first place. All these years living downtown, and I had never once ventured out to the river walkway—a colorful portrait of piers, pedestrians, and possibilities. Yet this wonderland was a mere four blocks from my apartment.

I suddenly felt like I had been socked in the stomach, and yet it was not the running cramps I was feeling. A powerful thought slipped into my consciousness: by staying in one place, I was missing everything. I let out one last long sigh, grabbed my loose waistband, and hobbled home. The next day, still wearing my ratty uncushioned sneakers, I ran a little further.

Eventually, I invested in new footwear and, for that matter, a new mindset. And although that ordinary day when everything seemed to change somehow started me down the running path, I still had my doubts.

I have to admit that I still hear a voice inside me telling me that people who run are those who have time to burn. Who in their right mind can afford to start off their day with a brisk jog, rather than a brittle meeting? For those working in social justice, the loud, menacing voice that screams, *We are trying to change the world, people!* is a common one, and sometimes that voice screams for a life of work, and work alone. That inner conversation hasn't ended, and I don't expect it ever will. Even these days, I constantly ask myself if I have the right to prioritize my running over an important email or deadline. And let's face it—sometimes that voice is coming more from reluctance to get out there than true devotion to work. In any case, it's a daily issue, coming up for me during that half-an-hour argument I have with myself each morning between waking up and leaving my apartment.

But then, through gritted teeth, I am eventually out the door, and it all makes sense once again. I channel my inner teenager and blast Patti LuPone music, or showtunes (my friend Sally, one of my running mentors, taught me that the soundtrack to *A Chorus Line* makes a perfect running companion). I leave my baggage at home (quite literally—most other times I am bogged down with heavy books and computers) and fly by the seat of my pants. I am light and anonymous. I zigzag through fast pedestrians and slow tourists, zip through the streets of lower Manhattan. I make mental notes of coffee places to visit, parks to take my dog, beautiful buildings to show my partner, Mariann. I zone out, drifting into the dramatic crescendo of "The Music and the Mirror" blasting through my earbuds, and suddenly I realize that I have run all the way uptown. I somehow remain unnoticed, untouched by the bustling gritty city around me. I play by own rules. I jump in puddles. I pee at Starbucks' bathrooms without buying anything. I say "beep beep" instead of "on your left" as I pass double strollers in Chelsea. I slow down long enough to pat the top of cute dogs' heads. Sometimes I skip.

It is often during a run—the fullest expression of my physical freedom—that I think of the billions of animals who are hidden in a dark world of unimaginable suffering, unfathomable cruelty, and unrelenting exploitation. As I run, I am free, but they are confined, utterly and completely. It is frequently the sight of a pigeon, an animal that is forever tattooed on my arm and Mariann's shoulder, that inspires me to reflect upon this hideous contrast.

These stunningly beautiful birds—who possess an iridescence that is unsurpassed by nearly any other creature—were brought to the United States by the Dutch as food animals. But the pigeons escaped this death trap, the food system. These days, they are loathed, considered dirty and irksome. Yet they persevere, unscathed, glorious reminders of what is possible when we try hard enough to get out, when we remain true to ourselves and our nature.

I like to believe that when these sweet birds were indeed "pigeonholed" as "food animals," they laughed commodification in the face and then got away. This mass exodus from animal agriculture is particularly meaningful to me, since the breadth of the work I do carries the ultimate goal of ending the exploitation of animals—

focusing in particular on the victims of animal agriculture. Pigeons escaped, even though they are still maligned. They are ambassadors, indifferent to an unsympathetic society that sneers at them. They are unintentional rabble-rousers.

Perhaps it's because of that that pigeons give me hope. I run as they fly; I stare at the sky as they soar. I look over the Hudson River as they whish and whoosh left and right, showing off in their glory. They are free. These birds represent to me all that is possible, and all that is still yet to be done.

Meanwhile, like these escapees, I leap. I am privileged, I am free. I am able-bodied, I am middle-class, I am not "without. . . ." My freedom as I jog through what I unabashedly call The Best City in the World works twofold for me: I recognize the privileges I have, and at the same time I see the unjust horror perpetrated upon those whose voices are squelched so readily. Those who are less lucky, for whatever reason. The animals—human and other—who either cannot run freely, or who, even if they are able, have no place to run but away.

And sometimes when I run, I confront sadness that does not pertain to animals at all—personal feelings I usually manage to suppress, except for during my early morning adventures. I tear up as I think about how my active, independent grandmother became wheelchair-bound and died. Or I sit in the regret of an argument I had with Mariann that morning, in which—I see now—I was wrong. I process, I pontificate, I pound the pavement. I laugh out loud, I cry out loud, I curse out loud. It's New York, so I do not seem any more nuts than the next guy.

For me, that is the connection between my animal rights activism, my commitment to veganism, and my running. I am a stronger activist not only because I build my body and energy through my running, but because of the time I have to reflect on the world. More than anything else, running has given me that time and space: time during which I can think more clearly than at any other moment during the day; space I share with nobody but myself on early mornings in the city, before the hot sun is fully ablaze, before the freezing cold snow has enveloped my neighborhood, or the unforgiving foot traffic has made it impossible to move. When I run, I realize that not only can I move, but I recognize that we, the world of people who care, can move mountains. Put simply, running allows me to appreciate what freedom is, and how precious it is.

I am not a runner. But when I run, after I fight myself not to, I experience a cathartic shift out of my everyday, to-do-list thinking. I see in my mind's eye the subjugated, the marginalized, the oppressed. I consciously juxtapose that mental image with images of liberation, and I allow them to fill and inspire me. With my new body, my new hope, my new conviction—which I rediscover daily—I connect to a world laden with sadness, and believe that just maybe I can change it a bit for the better.

When it comes to the connections between running and veganism, there are links I could easily come up with. I could tell you that it's important for vegans to be the embodiment and vision of good health, because if we don't look good, how are we going to "convert" those around us to a compassionate, animal-friendly way of life? I could tell you that the reason I run is because I feel "at one" with nature and wildlife, which fuels my animal advocacy. I could explain that I run because I want so badly to bash any nonsensical stereotype of vegans being poor athletes. Perhaps most importantly, I could make the argument that by impacting myself in a positive way through running, I can make myself a better activist, and then have an impact on others.

But, fundamentally, all of those reasons describe ways in which my running serves my veganism. And that is how it is for me. I am vegan because it is a moral imperative, a direct extension of my worldview, and because there is absolutely no way to justify exploiting animals, ever. I do not run because I find it a moral imperative, and I do not have any intention to "convert" those who choose not to run. Unlike the way I see veganism, I think running, or choosing not to, is a completely personal decision. It works for some people, and doesn't work for others. It's certainly not the only way to improve yourself or your health. And all sorts of activities can make you a better, stronger, happier, more thoughtful person, and, thus, a better activist. These might include adopting healthful habits, meditation, and, for some people (not me, particularly), spiritual practice. Like running, all those things are fantastic, if they work for you. But, unlike veganism, they do not directly reduce the harm one does to others.

So while you can indeed find overlaps between veganism and running, and in many ways they are both important, at the end of the day only one of them will truly impact others, while the other will just impact you. (Not that there's anything wrong with embracing health, or seeking reflection, or, for that matter, finding inner peace. I'm a fan of inner peace, actually; it's something I'm constantly on the lookout for. Occasionally, when I'm running through the Harlem Hills, or Battery Park City, I catch a glimpse of it, ever so slightly, and I run a little faster.)

I'm constantly aware that there are contradictions between the private, introspective, personally driven world of running, and the public, other-directed arena of activism. Yet, somehow, running helps me survive in this upside-down world—a world with such tremendous potential for goodness, but one that still allows greed to destroy everything that is precious. I am not a runner, but I will continue to run. Both on the ground, and in my heart, toward a vision permanently carved into my mind's eye, of what will be possible when we stop consuming animals and instead live according to a compassionate worldview in which nobody is harmed.

I doubt very much that my inability to think of myself as a runner will change, even despite the fact that, in 2012, I completed a half-marathon—a tiring yet deeply rewarding experience that temporarily took over my personality and schedule. I've no doubt I will run in another long race. I will cheer when I see another participant alongside me touting a "No Meat Athlete" T-shirt, or maybe some knee-high compression socks that say "Vegan"—like the ones I wear. We'll be united, that fellow racer and I. We'll share a moment of understanding, sisterhood, comradeship, insanity, plant-based power, commitment. Maybe that fellow vegan racer will not be a runner, either. Maybe, instead, she'll be playing the part of one, as I do. Just a grown-up kid from New Jersey who one day decided to ditch meat, dairy, and eggs: a decision that shaped the story of the rest of her life, and the next day found herself lacing up her sneakers; a decision that remains a day-to-day commitment.

My running gave me the ability to see myself as someone who

moves, but, beyond that, it gave me an opportunity to constantly prioritize what's important to me, and for me. Each time I run, the kind of thoughts and experiences I can somehow have only when I am moving help me to reshape my understanding of a world that is still so mysterious to me—so breathtakingly beautiful and heart-breakingly sad at the same time. Somehow, when I run, I navigate the sidewalk cracks in such a way that they are no longer something I fear, but rather, something I expect—little challenges put there for me to tackle. Sometimes I will trip on them, but I will always eventually find my *get up and go*.

That is why I run. Not to change the world *per se*—even though I want very much to be a part of that change, and I will not settle for anything less than a new world that's free of suffering—but because if I don't run, then how I will ever get anywhere? Even a non-runner such as myself can understand how important it is to move, whether toward a finish line or toward the future.

Special thanks to Mariann Sullivan and Gena Hamshaw.

12

Three Days

Scott Spitz

DAY 1

The surgeon said a lot this morning. *Malignant. Growth. Concerning. Fluids. Rupture.*

It was more in *how* he said it, than *what* exactly. His tone had changed from our first meeting, where he seemed clinical, robotic, routine. This time, he entered the room with a nurse at his side, a smile on his face that seemed just a touch too forced, and an inflection that was reaching, struggling for words that hit their mark, but not too pointedly. He was saying something without actually saying it.

"I found something in the CT scan I wasn't expecting to see. . . . You actually don't have a hernia, but something more problematic. . . . There are cells that are reproducing, secreting a mucus . . . continuing to grow . . . extending from the appendix and potentially rupturing the abdomen and filling the surrounding area with mucus cells. . . . Extensive operation that involves a blast of chemo. . . ."

Again, there was so much said, but something not being said. Unfazed by the news I thought I was hearing, I questioned the surgeon, and he replied, "Well, these cells that rupture from the appendix, we *do* consider them cancerous."

And he said it . . . I thought. He said "Cancer*ous*," not "Cancer." I never heard him say, "You. Have. Stomach. Cancer." He just used words like "tumor," "malignant," "chemo," "cancer*ous*." I certainly didn't want to go back to my parents or anyone else saying I had stomach cancer when I actually didn't. Maybe I had something that *could* be stomach cancer. Maybe I had something that could turn *into* stomach cancer. Maybe they needed to run more tests?

But why was the surgeon speaking in broken medical English? Why did I get the feeling he was being intentionally nicer to me than he was last time? Why did a nurse have to be present? Why was I scheduled to see an oncologist to set up an operation?

I left the exam room and shook his hand goodbye. Then I shook the nurse's hand. She took mine in hers and instead of a formal parting, she placed her other hand on top, like a protective cradle, holding it longer than is normative, and said, "Take care. Call me with any questions you may have."

I got it. She wasn't just there as a witness, a nurse in training. She was there to *console* me. Yeah, I got it. They just told me I had stomach cancer. The doctor was trying to deliver what is intense, potentially life-changing news with the greatest of care and compassion he could muster. She was there as the human face of medicine, the support structure. She was there for *me*, should I need it.

I paid the visit fee with the last remaining portion of my credit card that the maximum would allow and started walking to my car, absorbing the realization that, yes, I was just told I have stomach cancer. Me. Stomach cancer. Me. Cancer.

Wait, who are we talking about here again? Me? Seriously? I'm supposed to internalize the fact that I have stomach cancer? I'm supposed to put those two words together without hesitation? I've suddenly entered the Culture of Cancer? But there must be some mistake. Maybe you didn't see my epic run last week, you know, where I knocked out thirty trail miles at a seven-minute-per-mile pace? That's not something a cancer patient does. What just happened here?

Cancer is not a part of my identity. Cancer is something my grandmother died from years ago. Cancer is something I watched kill my sister. Cancer is something that happens to other people. Or older people. Or . . . wait, what just happened here, again? I was supposed to have had a simple umbilical hernia. I was supposed to be scheduling a basic operation to put everything back in place and have me attacking my marathon personal best in just a couple of hopeful weeks. I was supposed to be looking forward to eliminating that confusing feeling of bloat and pain around my abdomen. I was supposed to be setting an example of effort and discipline for my son. I wasn't supposed to be leaving the hospital as another cancer statistic. That was *serious*.

But life is nothing if not an unpredictable adventure. And I have a . . . a . . . I don't even know what I have. A *diagnosis*, I guess. A further understanding of the pain and prior symptoms I'd been experiencing for the past couple of months. A deep and continuous examination of, well, life in general. The immediate present, a bit of the past, and an incredibly uncertain future. I just have my thoughts, really. Coupled with a continuing feeling of discomfort in my abdomen, too, I guess. What I *don't* have is a new identity.

I *don't* have a cancer identity and I don't *want* a cancer identity.

This may change I suppose. But that feels awkward. I honestly don't want to be that guy with cancer. I don't want to be that guy overcoming invasive surgery and a continued chemotherapy plan. I don't want to be that guy that ran and is trying to get back to running after cancer. I don't want any part of that.

I'm that vegan runner. That's who I am. That's what I *feel* like. Even though I'm not currently running, that's what I feel like. This new diagnosis, this is just another stupid obstacle thrown in my path, much like the injury I had in my weakened right leg in 2011. Much like the break I took to concentrate on my personal life. Much like the nerve pain that sidelined me just before winter this year. That's all this is, just another stupid obstacle I need to get out of the way so I can get back to throwing down mile repeats and epic long runs on the trails of Brown County.

My coach responded to the news, "The Scott Spitz story has taken another twist. Beat this motherfucker and then please be boring for a while." He gets it. This is just part of the story. Though there will be no "being boring for a while" once we get past this part. I assured him, "There are roads and trails being unrun as we speak!"

A Little on Perspective
I harbor a specific approach towards veganism and health, which openly negates the "magic bullet" of optimum health and long life that some

try to ascribe to veganism. There are those that tout the health benefits of veganism in a way that leads others to believe that if they stop eating animal products they will be free from any concerns regarding sickness and disease. This is patently false and I do my part to make this known at every opportunity. Can veganism aid you in combating disease? Yes. Can veganism help alleviate many sicknesses? Yes. Can veganism help reverse certain afflictions? Yes. But does this mean eating vegan turns your body bulletproof, stops heart attacks, reverses diabetes, guarantees weight loss, and makes cancer a non-issue? No. No. And no. We only do a disservice to ourselves and the animals we seek to liberate by exaggerating the health claims of veganism and leading people to believe in an outcome that is disproven by every healthy eating, active, living vegan that develops, say, cancer of any stripe.

When I told my friends my news, I was inundated with supportive responses, expressing an equal disbelief that someone who is consistently physically active as myself, who doesn't eat meat or dairy, who eats minimal refined sugars, who eats primarily whole grains and whole foods, who pays attention to their diet and makes an effort to eat in ways that suggest optimal health, can still get a life-threatening disease. Admittedly, it doesn't seem fair . . . but life isn't fair. Life is physical. There is no morality in the seeds that sprout from the ground. There is no justice in the winds that blow across the earth. There is no great sense of ethics that spins the planets in orbit. There is merely a realization of the greatest chance and circumstance to ever enter our lives, a constantly changing and evolving physical existence, a completely *imperfect* order that seeks to correct itself continuously. And we are just a part of that. Or in other words, *shit happens.* Sometimes smokers live to 103. Sometimes healthy people have abnormalities. Sometimes health-conscious vegans get cancer. That's just how it goes. And the sooner we accept this, the more comforted we are when the chance and circumstance of life turn on us.

I'm glad I never followed the stream of wishful thinking and put it out there that I was bulletproof. I'm not. I live my life consciously, making decisions that benefit me physically and mentally to the utmost degree, and even though the forces of chance and imperfection just smacked me in the face, every conscious decision I made to this point and onward is worth it. That's what ultimately matters. Not that we "succeed" in life by avoiding the plagues and diseases of our time, but that we simply try, doing everything in our power to benefit both ourselves and others.

As much as before, go vegan!

DAY 2

This morning I ran errands essentially canceling parts of my life. I drove to my job and officially quit, as I was assured that I was "going to be out of work for quite some time" and the recovery wasn't going to be quick. I didn't have insurance at this job and my employers weren't going to be able to wait out an extended recovery. They were absolutely great about it and offered me references and a position upon return should I need it. Of course, this now leaves me without both income and insurance, which is probably the most precarious place one can find oneself in, in the face of intensive medical procedures.

Leaving my job, I drove to my coach's athletic store and dropped off a massage ball he gave me to test and review and turned in my racing singlet. I'm not gonna lie, that stings; but it was a matter of logistics. Someone currently racing will need it and I'll just pick up another when I return. I assured my coach that returning the items was not a gesture of quitting, but just not taking something and giving nothing back. I promised my coach that I'd be back to pick up that singlet on the other side.

It was then a short ride to the YMCA to cancel my membership and save the monthly payment, as I wasn't going to be able to use their services until my body was ready again. I assured them it was nothing they did, and although they offered a sixty-day hold, I said I was pretty sure I was going to be out for more than sixty days.

And yet, even with an abrupt halting of my daily routines, that I rinsed and repeated day in and day out, without an end in sight, nothing seems different. I have this *thing* . . . and it's not very real. I'm just dealing with it and going about my days, almost as if I'm just waiting for it to go away so I can get back to running again, sort of like I handled most of my past injuries.

It is, of course, not going away. And it must be dealt with or I'll never run again.

So maybe right now, the gap of time between now and the operation, is preventing me from recognizing that things *are* different. Or at least that they *will* be different. I know they will, but unfortunately I don't know *how* they will be different. And until I pose my questions to the right people and get sufficient answers, it's going to be hard to see how things are different, though, admittedly, I should probably get on that as soon as possible so the shock of my previous life and (temporary) new life to come isn't so great.

Pretty soon though, I think the weight of this is going to come crashing down and *everything* will be different. But hey, I'll be prepared. I've got a near army of friends and acquaintances and strangers coming out of the woodwork offering help, services, guidance, and encouragement—so much that it's a little overwhelming and I'm struggling to accept their generosity, in part because everything still seems the same and I feel undeserving of resources I know are not easy to part with. I guess sooner or later I should recognize that things may seem the same, but they certainly aren't. This might just be the calm before the storm.

Whatever is coming though, it's going to be dealt with—because I have running to get back to.

Not Running

Pseudomyxoma peritonei (PMP) is a very rare type of cancer that usually begins in your appendix as a small growth, called a polyp. Or, more rarely, it can start in other parts of the bowel, the ovary or bladder. This polyp eventually spreads through the wall of your appendix and spreads cancerous cells to the lining of the abdominal cavity (the peritoneum). These cancerous cells produce mucus, which collects in the abdomen as a jelly-like fluid called mucin.

We don't know what causes this type of cancer. Most cancers are caused by a number of different factors working together.

This description sounds relatively tame, but the greater problems involve the cancer growing and the accumulation of mucin in the abdominal area, effectively putting increasing pressure upon the abdominal organs. It's hard to determine exactly what damage has been done to any internal organs until the operation begins and the organs can be viewed directly, which may entail the removal of said organs (appendix, gall bladder, spleen). In the interim, however, the mucin creates an overall feeling of both bloat and pressure, so even minor jostling of the abdomen/core gives discomfort and pain.

Before I had a more accurate diagnostic theory, and before I understood the actual process of what was going on inside me, I was in agony and very limited in my movement. I was having a terrible time sleeping at night as any position involved great pain and pressure. I was walking slightly bent over, trying to cradle and protect my abdomen, taking the most gingerly steps down stairs or off curbs. Driving was problematic as I braced for every bump in the road. Putting any food in my system would bring on near immediate pains moving throughout my abdomen as the food made its way through my intestines. I was, rather quickly, a physical mess.

But then I figured out what was going on. I recognized the mass and mucin in my belly were at such an extent that all my organs were under continuous pressure, so any time I put food into me, I was essentially pushing back on that pressure and causing the pains and limited mobility. Initially, I was eating full-on meals like normal, mimicking my past eating habits that centered around fueling for longer runs, so the amount of food I was taking in was causing intense pressure and putting me into near debilitating pain, especially at night when my stomach was already full from eating throughout the day.

And so I changed all that. Very quickly I started eating less, switched almost entirely to easily chewed and digested foods and ate them in small portions, as if in grazing mode. Breakfast is now quite minimal, bananas are my best friend, and I'm trying to eat nutrient-dense foods that pack it all in small portions. If I do slip up and eat more at night than I should, I pay the price the next day. Overall, it's not my preferred way of eating, but the benefit of not walking around in pain is totally worth it.

So, I'm not running. But it's different this time. It's serious. So I can handle it. This is not a confusing injury I'm just waiting to heal itself so I can get back out there and put in work. This time it's a "condition" that not only won't heal on its own, but will actually get worse, and I know what is needed to "fix" it, to get back to functioning health, and to then get back to running. Because yes, I'm getting back to running. That's all I can see . . . a void of my life post-operation, that at some point entails getting back to running, hard and fast. I don't know when and I don't care what unsatisfactory timelines might be offered to me, at some point, I'm going to run again.

I am not running right now. I can't. That is the bad news. The good news is, I can see through the void, and off in the distance I'm growing smaller and smaller.

DAY 3

My son should not have an intimate knowledge of cancer. He's *six*.

When I picked him up in Charleston, West Virginia, last Saturday for a visit during his spring break, I quickly explained to him that I was going to be put in a machine that would take a picture of the insides of my body. I asked him if he wanted to watch, thinking that might be pretty fascinating for a boy his age, but also wanting him to have a direct experience with modern medicine and technology. I think he would have actually enjoyed watching, but the walkie-talkies the Easter Bunny dropped off held more appeal.

Little did I know that that machine was gathering images of something far more serious than the suspected hernia around my navel. When I met with the surgeon the next day and was given the news I was by myself. My first thought was to call my dad and let him know, allowing him to pass the information to my mom in a way I trusted he would do best. Then I sat in the car for a few minutes to do a little processing, in the midst of realizing I needed to find a way to talk to my son about this.

When I arrived back at my parents', my dad was already on the computer researching PMP and my mom seemed to be doing okay. My son was playing in the other room by himself. I didn't say anything initially, but sat with him and watched a little TV, just enjoying the comfort of his snuggling. I knew I should tell him soon though, because the conversations that were going to begin would not be missed by his little, hyperactive ears.

I sat him on the couch to give the info to him directly, initially struggling to find the right way to describe the specifics in a way a six-year-old could understand.

"You know how Papa's stomach has been hurting him? Well, the photos they took of my inside yesterday showed the doctor something we didn't think it was. Now, I want you to know I'm not 'sick,' but I just have a problem inside my stomach that needs to be fixed. It's called a cancer. There are these cells that are growing and causing problems in my belly, making everything hurt, and I'm

going to need to get them out of there. It's a pretty serious problem
and if I don't take care of this, I can die from it, but that's why we
took the pictures of my inside and talked to the doctor. When we
meet with the next doctor we are going to set up an appointment
to get rid of the bad cells inside of me. Does that make sense? And
I know this can be confusing, so if you have any questions about
this, you can ask me anything, okay? Ask me anything you want if
you get confused."

He wrinkled his nose and fidgeted during my explanation, but
paid direct attention and expressed genuine interest. He paused a
moment after I finished, then asked, "So you could die from this?"

It was obvious the most extreme element of my explanation had
made an impression.

"Well, if we didn't take care of it, yes, I could."

"Whoooaaa," he said, with a six-year-old's fascination.

"But that's why we are going to take care of it. That's why we are
going to the doctor's to get everything fixed. And remember, you
can ask me any questions about this if you want, you just let me
know, okay?"

We got up from the chairs and went back to making lunch and getting ready to eat. Ten minutes later, I finished making the sandwiches,
walked into the dining room to check something on my computer,
and found him sitting at the table, his arms crossed and chin resting
on his hands, just looking off pensively . . . *very* unlike him.

"Hey, buddy . . . are you okay?"

"Yeah," he calmly said.

"Remember, if you have any questions about this, you can ask
me," I assured him.

In hindsight, I was so glad he was here to experience this development right along with me, getting a very direct knowledge of being given this sort of news. That way, any explanation I gave him was fully understandable, instead of trying to convey this over the phone from hundreds of miles away. I was there all week to give him the straight story if needed.

But what I didn't realize until later was that, even more importantly, it wasn't how I described it to him, or that I was there to answer his questions, but that he was there to absorb everything going around him with his keen six-year-old perception. He got to see the way in which my family reacted to the news. He got to see how my friends reacted. He got to see the love and care everyone extended to me as we spent our time around the city. And he got to see how I was able to process, accept, and make the best of the new awareness. And that has to have the deepest effect on him in the immediate sense and in the future. This may be more valuable to his future than either of us can ever imagine right now. So for this cancer to make itself known during the very week he was visiting was immeasurably lucky, and I'm so grateful he was here to share the experience with me.

But I don't mean to romanticize this. I wish to hell he didn't have to experience this at all, nor me.

I walked him towards the coffee shop in Charleston for the drop-off this afternoon, stopping briefly outside for a final hug, to say goodbye and address the experience one more time, letting him know that I was going to be in the hospital soon and the next time we Skyped it might actually be from the hospital, "which will be pretty neat, huh?"

I told him I loved him and we walked into the store, but suddenly he uncharacteristically stopped, not beelining it straight towards his mama. He turned to me.

"Papa. Will you call me and tell me if your cancer goes away?"

"Of *course* I will. Absolutely. I'll call you and tell you how everything is going and let you know exactly when it goes away, okay?"

And with that he was appeased, running off to his mama and back to North Carolina.

Now it's time to buckle down and face what's coming.

13

Striving for Peace in Every Step

Catherine Berlot

Each step is a miracle.
Each step is healing.
Each step is nourishing.
Each step is freedom.

—THICH NHAT HANH,
FROM *PEACE IS EVERY BREATH*

On a beautiful sunny Saturday morning in April, I decide to go for a nine-mile run in the part of rural central Pennsylvania that I call home. The snow flurries that were predicted a few days earlier have never materialized, and it is now in the mid thirties, with a fresh breeze. The purple, yellow, and white crocuses outside my kitchen window are blooming, promising that longer and warmer days are on the way. As I set off for my run, I note that they will soon be joined by daffodils, hyacinths, peonies, and bleeding hearts. Similarly, the redbud trees across the street are almost ready to become lacy pink clouds. Robins and cardinals are out and about.

I start heading east and then uphill. Since I'm just warming up, this is a bit challenging, but the reward is that I get an increasingly impressive view of a valley carpeted with fields of corn, wheat, and soybeans and neighboring forested hills as I climb higher. There follows an exhilarating downhill stretch under cover of plenty of trees with a stream on the left. At the foot of the hill I turn onto a secluded and canopied road, still accompanied by the soothing sight and sound of the stream.

Then I get to a junction and the smell of the pig farm down the intersecting road hits me. For those of you who haven't experienced it, the smell of a pig farm can be overwhelming. The acrid ammonia gets into your throat and your eyes tear up, making it hard to concentrate on anything else. And this is only what you encounter outside. What the pigs themselves must endure continuously is obviously orders of magnitude worse.

I have never smelled the farm before. It must be some trick of the wind, or perhaps the barn is being cleaned out. Since the barn is set back from the road, I have never seen it up close. Occasionally, one or two pigs will actually be outside, between the building and the road. Are they the somewhat luckier ones? I have, however, heard the pigs before. Their heartrending screams made my blood run cold. What was happening to them? Were they being castrated without anesthesia? Were they having their tails cut off? Were they being slaughtered, perhaps by what is known in the industry as "PACing" (Pounding Against Concrete)? Since this is a breeding farm, was the distress coming from mothers being transferred from gestation crates to farrowing crates, or being separated from their babies, or from babies who were considered unviable being killed?

Today, the smell is just as bad as the screams. I can feel my muscles tightening, but I concentrate on the sound of the gentle stream and keep going.

IN THE PAST, my anger led to tense muscles that worked against one another and made running more of an effort. This mindset was counterproductive for both my running and my burgeoning vegan activism. At my lowest point, my stride became so heavy and unbalanced that I was wearing out my running shoes in a very peculiar way. I couldn't seem to stop "kicking" the road as I swung my left leg forward. It wasn't that I was trying to take out my frustrations on the road. It was just those tight muscles getting worn out. And anyway, the road was winning. The front medial side of my left shoe (Saucony Progrid Ride 2) wore all the way through. I went back to the running store, owned by a physical therapist, and showed her my shoe, hoping she might have an idea of why this was happening. But she'd never seen anything like this form of damage and was so impressed that she pulled out her cell phone and took a picture to show to the sales rep the next time he stopped by.

My anger and accompanying gait problems are now subsiding as I take to heart the teachings of Vietnamese Zen Buddhist monk Thich Nhat Hanh. I discovered his work after I had become vegan. I wanted to find a spiritual tradition that embraces all animals, human and nonhuman alike, as beings, and in which actions are consistent with the teachings. Not every Buddhist is vegan or even vegetarian, although the teachings of Buddhism, if actually applied to life, would seem to say that ethical veganism is an essential part of being a Buddhist.

Nhat Hanh (the "Thich" is an honorific) is nonetheless a very vegan-friendly Buddhist. He has devoted his life to generating peace and reconciliation through what he calls "Engaged Buddhism." He actively promoted peace during the Vietnam War without taking sides, and as a consequence was denied permission to return to Vietnam for many years. Because of his anti-war efforts, Martin Luther King nominated him for the Nobel Peace Prize in 1967. He has established numerous Buddhist practice centers around the world and lives in one of them, Plum Village in France.

Thich Nhat Hanh's teachings emphasize "interbeing," "non-self," and impermanence. We "interare" in that we are all connected with one another regardless of race, sex, or species. We are "empty" of a separate self because we all contain elements of each other. We must live in the moment, because we and the world around us are impermanent. The present moment is all we have, but that is not a bad thing. We can make every moment wonderful. Nhat Hanh is very concerned about the environmental consequences of our actions and frequently cites animal consumption as being a major contributor to worldwide hunger and climate change.

I'm finding that I can alter my reality by changing the way I think, which has useful applications for both running and vegan activism. Nhat Hanh has a lot to say about walking meditation and I have taken the liberty of applying his thoughts to running rather than walking. Some of the ideas I meditate on while running, adapted from his guided meditations on walking in his book *The Long Road Turns to Joy*, are as follows, where I substitute the word *run* for *walk*:

Walk as if you are kissing the Earth with your feet, as if you are massaging the Earth with each step.

Visualize a lotus, a tulip, or a gardenia blooming under each step the moment your foot touches the ground. If you practice beautifully like this, your friends will see fields of flowers everywhere you walk.

The miracle is to walk on Earth. . . . The Earth is a miracle. Each step is a miracle. Taking steps on our beautiful planet can bring real happiness. As you walk, be fully aware of your foot, the ground, and the connection between them, which is your conscious breathing.

We walk for ourselves, and we walk for those who cannot walk. We walk for all living beings—past, present, and future.

Thinking like this has gone a long way towards making running more relaxing. It makes me feel like both the road and I are getting a massage. Currently I'm running in Mizuno Wave Rider 15s and have yet to ruin them with my previous wear pattern. It could be that these shoes are virtually indestructible, but I like to think that my attitude and stride have changed, too.

————

PROCEEDING WEST, I pass two horses who seem content to graze beside a lily pad–filled pond. They calmly watch me go by. I start to relax and breathe more easily as I head up another uphill stretch bordered by trees and accompanied by another stream. However, my reward at the top is not an excellent view, but the sign for a farm that advertises "grass-fed meat" along with the picture of a smiling cow. Really? I didn't know that "meat" could eat anything. In the distance, I can see some of the grazing cows. They seem happy enough right now, but they aren't living at a farmed animal sanctuary where they can live out their natural lives in peace. At some point, when they are barely out of infancy, they will be loaded onto a trailer and taken to the same kind of slaughterhouse in which feedlot cattle are killed.

I go all out down the hill. Midway is a house with a sign over the garage that proclaims "Deer Hunters Point." This route is not runnable during the two weeks right after Thanksgiving, when the Pennsylvania deer hunting rifle season opens. Hunters in camouflage and carrying high-tech rifles can be seen hiking by the side of the road. I believe it is illegal to shoot from the road, but I'm not interested in taking any chances, so I stay away during that time. Right before the season starts, I see a lot of deer in the early mornings on my runs. They are all gone after those two weeks.

Now the road crosses the stream. I catch my breath and continue on a flat stretch until I come to a gravel road that rises through some beautiful woods with a river running down a gully on the right. As I emerge from the woods, I can see a chicken shed across the gully. Although I've never seen inside of it, I can imagine that the chickens are packed so tightly into cages that they can hardly move and have no room to spread their wings. Instead of being able to hatch a reasonable number of babies and raise them lovingly, these chickens are doomed to lay an egg almost every day until they are "spent," at which time they will be hauled off in the transport truck that drives right by my house, on their way to be slaughtered. Their bodies will probably be bought up by the USDA for school lunch, military, and prison programs, because these poor animals are so fragile there isn't much of a market for them otherwise.

Compare the lives of these invisible birds to those of the wild turkeys that live nearby. Once, I saw a wild turkey mom and her babies fly into the trees in full view of the shed. I tell the chickens, as I always do, that I love them and am bearing witness to their suffering.

At the top of the road is a church. Many times I'm either inspired or amused by the slogans displayed on the message boards of the churches in this area, such as "THE BEST WAY TO ESCAPE A PROBLEM IS TO SOLVE IT" OR "SIGN BROKEN. COME INSIDE FOR MESSAGE" OR "WHAT'S MISSING IN CH_ _ CH? U R." However, I find it upsetting when they advertise a "chicken and waffles" dinner, a meat-centric community potluck, or an "ice cream social." How can a religion that is supposed to be about love and compassion sanction the abuse and killing of innocent beings for consumption? Today, the message is "DAILY EXERCISE IS GOOD FOR YOU. WALK WITH JESUS TODAY." I take a few deep breaths and focus on how running is good for me and that I am running for the animals. Then I continue on my way.

MY NEW WAY of thinking is not only making me relax and improving my speed and endurance, but it's changing my reaction to animal abuse from anger to sorrow, compassion, and a determined resolve to be a more resilient and effective animal advocate. Now, even when I'm struggling while I'm running, I'm grateful to be able to run freely. I think often about my nonhuman sisters and brothers who live miserable lives of confinement before being killed at a young age. I run for them as well as myself. I send love and prayers to the abused animals I pass. I think of those who can't spread their wings or turn around while I'm lucky enough to be able to work on my running technique.

One aspect of running technique that I'm working on is timing, getting the various muscles to fire in the right order so that they can work together in harmony. Timing is important for animal advocacy, too, in that different liberation strategies may be more effective at particular times and in particular contexts. We should be flexible and stay open to whatever works, rather than being caught up in images of what kinds of animal advocates we are. This process of "non-identification" strengthens patience, and we certainly need patience to be animal advocates. As I learn to recruit my core muscles so that I don't overwork my hamstrings and to relax my back so that it contributes just the right amount of effort, I'm striving to be more relaxed overall and to get out of my own way. In my communications with non-vegans, I'm finding that a more relaxed and patient attitude makes it easier to listen and ask questions so as to understand where they're coming from and to try to tailor my conversation accordingly.

On one run, I had just emerged from a charming old covered bridge and was passing by a field when I encountered a hunter.

"Do you know who owns this field?" he called out. "Do you

think they would mind if I shot a big gobbler that's over there, behind those trees?"

I certainly knew that I would mind. I would have liked to tell him how cruel and barbaric it would be to murder an innocent turkey, but I restrained myself.

"I don't know the owners," I replied. "But I don't think they would want you to trespass."

"I guess you have a point," he conceded. "The property is posted and I wouldn't want someone to hunt on my own land."

Amazingly enough, without further ado, he got back into his pickup truck and left without killing the turkey. Perhaps it was a lesson that not expressing and amplifying my anger in a tirade against hunting was the most productive thing I could do for that particular animal.

When I first went vegan, it wasn't all about me, but it was more so than it is now. The focus was on *my* reactions to animal cruelty and *my* decision that *I* wasn't going to continue to be a part of the systems that perpetrated animal abuse. Similarly, I went running to work off *my* frustrations and because I loved the way it made *me* feel. Now I'm learning to see that I am not a separate self, to understand that I'm connected with all other beings. Similar to the idea of "Engaged Buddhism," I am working to evolve into an "engaged running vegan." I am not just running for myself. For me, this means learning to find ways to be an animal advocate while I'm running.

I now see all my runs as a potential means of outreach to change people's hearts and minds. Whereas once I was annoyed when cars crowded me on the roads, now I try to see each passing one as an opportunity for activism. Often, when I run I wear one of the many jerseys that I've received from participating in Vegan Outreach's Team Vegan fundraising campaigns. The slogan on the back, "Go Vegan Go," can be interpreted both as a call to the observer to go vegan as well as encouragement for the running vegan (me) to keep on running. I'm not sure if the drivers can read my shirts, but I hope some of them can and may perhaps be inspired that a person can be vegan and fit enough to be a runner. I also welcome my infrequent encounters with pedestrians, usually those walking their dogs, who are more likely to have time to read my shirts. I smile and say a friendly *hello* as I go by, hoping to counteract any stereotypes they may have about judgmental vegans.

I TURN LEFT and run down and then uphill. A little further on, a mile from home, is a volunteer fire company. I'm glad to have them so close to home in case of an emergency, but it saddens me that they sell gun-raffle tickets and host turkey-shoot fundraisers. I run east for my final mile. If I went another mile, I would pass a back-yard small-scale factory farm that holds a never-ending succession of doomed animals: two calves chained inside a tent, a tethered goat and her baby, short-lived flocks of chickens. The only "perma-nent" animal is an old black dog, who probably wonders why he hasn't yet been taken away or killed.

Learning to transform my vegan anger into constructive activ-ism and to teach my muscles to work together in harmony as I run has been a challenging, but ultimately rewarding experience. I like to think that eventually the hearts and minds of those who have yet to develop compassion for nonhuman animals will be awakened. Only then, while out running in this more compassionate world, will I encounter pigs, cows, and chickens who are living happy natural lives in sanctuaries. Farms will advertise fresh organic produce with pictures of happy and healthy children picking their own vegetables. The churches will have signs saying things like "WHAT HAVE YOU DONE TODAY TO SPREAD LOVE AND COMPASSION TO ALL YOUR FELLOW EARTHLINGS?"

The journey is certainly not over, but meditations such as this "Walking Meditation" (also from *Peace Is Every Breath*) by Thich Nhat Hanh, keep me running in peace:

> The mind can go in a thousand directions,
> But on this beautiful path, I walk in peace.
> With each step, a gentle wind blows.
> With each step, a flower blooms.

14

What It Means to Be a Runner

Matt Frazier

Plenty of people who run, marathoners even, will tell you they're not really runners. There's no shortage of posts from running bloggers claiming they don't deserve the title, despite logging thirty or fifty or more miles every week.

For me, it took six marathons and qualifying for the Boston Marathon before I began to think of myself as a runner. But now that I'm comfortable with the name, I understand that being a runner has absolutely nothing to do with achievement. Rather, it's a mindset, a sense of connection with other runners . . . something that you just feel. You feel it when you pass the same runner, day in and day out on your little neighborhood loop, and exchange that almost imperceptible nod that says, *I understand.* You feel it when you're in the car and you drive by a runner laboring to get her day's miles in, and you wish that your little tap on the horn and thumbs-up could somehow express to her, *I know exactly what you're feeling, I've been there. Come on! You can get through it.*

And you felt it on April 15, 2013—Patriots' Day, Marathon Monday, our sport's proudest day—when you heard that something had gone horribly wrong at the Boston Marathon.

I think you become a runner when you recognize, in your own running, the essential kernel that motivates you and every other runner to get outside and log in the miles at the expense of so much else. Some runners do it for the medals and the T-shirts. Some run just to stay in shape. And others do it because, as they say, running is cheaper than therapy. But I think that at the most basic level, every one of us who runs does so because, deep down, we crave that little daily battle—against busyness, distraction, adversity, self-doubt—that every time we lace up our shoes, push ourselves out the door, and run, we win. And when you reach the point when you look at another runner and sense that he understands the ins and outs of the very same struggle you do—and that, whatever his method, he manages to win it, over and over, just like you—you feel the connection.

To me, that's what it means to be a runner.

When I got the text message that day in April 2013 that said there had been explosions at the finish line of the Boston Marathon, it was just about time for my scheduled five-miler. But as I watched the news with my wife (also a runner) and it steadily became apparent that this tragedy was no accident, I lost any motivation I had to run. Something about running felt selfish . . . or maybe I just understood that, no matter how well I ran, there would be no win that day.

For most of the afternoon, I simply wanted to forget. To forget that no big city marathon, especially not our beloved Boston Marathon, would ever be the same. To forget that the very phrase "Boston Marathon," with all the majesty and history and charm that are inextricably wrapped up within it, would be for many years supplanted by "Boston Marathon bombing," words that would recall the images of the bloody sidewalk and the videos of flashing lights, smoke, and panic. And for a few minutes, I wanted to forget that I was a runner at all. As if distancing myself from it all would help to numb the pain.

But as the evening wore on and tragic details continued to trickle in, I felt something I'd never felt before in my years as a runner: I sensed that I *had* to run . . . not for myself, but for someone—or some*thing*—else. To say that I ran to honor the victims would feel phony—when I headed out to run, I didn't know who they were or how old they were. All I could really guess was that each of the victims was either a runner, or someone who loved a runner. And while it didn't feel like it was my place to say that I was running for people I didn't know, as I ran during the last hour of daylight, I got the distinct sense that I was running for something I did know—deeply, and personally.

I was running, really, for running.

I longed to see just one other runner, someone with whom to share that familiar, subtle nod that would say, *I understand*, but mean so much more this time. In the whole hour, I didn't see a single other runner. But I knew they were out there, and that any who were would be thinking and feeling the same things I was. And that, of course, is again what it means to be a runner.

After I got home and my wife and I hugged our son extra tightly before putting him to bed, I signed onto Twitter, to connect with the community of runners I am lucky to have there.

I was unprepared for what awaited. There were hundreds of uplifting messages—quotes like Kathrine Switzer's, "If you are losing faith in humanity, go out and watch a marathon." Posts from runners who said that earlier in the day they had questioned their goal to one day run a marathon, but now felt more strongly than ever that they *had* to make it happen. News that everyone would be wearing a running shirt the day after, Boston gear if they had it, in a show of unity. And of course, the outpouring of support for the victims and their loved ones, the city of Boston, and the runners, many of whom were still in their running clothes and without a place to stay, their flights cancelled and their bags lost in the commotion. Without a place to stay, that is, until others stepped up and offered to help.

And when I went to bed, after a day that lasted far too long, I felt something I didn't expect to feel. Comfort. I was proud—and above all, grateful—to call myself a runner.

15

A Body in the Park

Martin Rowe

On December 29, 2013, the body of a man was discovered in Prospect Park, Brooklyn, New York, and rushed to Methodist Hospital on Seventh Avenue in Park Slope. He was dressed in running gear, carried an asthma inhaler, and had no identification on him. For several days, he lay in the hospital's intensive care unit, unknown. A photo of the runner in his hospital bed, his head heavily bandaged and encased in tubes, was issued to the media. Local running institutions, including JackRabbit Sports store, New York Road Runners, NYCRuns, and Prospect Park Track Club, circulated the photo, asking members if they recognized him. A friend who knew I often ran in Prospect Park sent me the image, but the angle of the shot and the medical paraphernalia around the man's head made it hard for me to identify him.

On January 7, 2014, the jogger's half-brother Charles identified the man. He was Rynn Berry, long-time vegan activist, historian, and author of, among other books, *Famous Vegetarians and Their*

Favorite Recipes and *Food for the Gods: Vegetarianism and the World's Religions.* He was sixty-eight years old. The face that had been unfamiliar to me was now impossible *not* to recognize: *Of course it was Rynn! How could it have been anyone else?* When I saw him, comatose, in the hospital the next day, his breathing and heartbeat regular, it seemed incredible, even shameful, that I hadn't immediately recognized him from the photo.

I was a welter of emotion. I'd known Rynn for more than twenty years. He contributed several articles and interviews to *Satya,* the magazine I cofounded with Beth Gould in 1994. Over the years, as we, writers and publishers both, circled each other (sometimes warily, but I like to believe, with mutual respect) Rynn took in stride my suggestion that he supply an introductory chapter for each interview in *Food for the Gods*—thus doubling his workload. When he asked me to write an introduction to *Hitler: Neither Vegetarian Nor Animal Lover,* and I produced a long piece designed to bulk up the monograph, he didn't complain that I questioned whether Hitler's diet really affected any serious person's notions about the moral basis of vegetarianism.

For the first eight years of its existence, my publishing company's offices overlooked Union Square in Manhattan. Every Wednesday and Saturday at the greenmarket, one could come across Rynn, standing at his table, his head-covering appropriate to the weather, purveying to the public *The Vegan Guide to New York City* and other works, and offering to append to their purchase an elegantly cursive dedication in best Indian ink. I loved that other aspect of Rynn: the reticent hustler, the retiring individual absolutely dedicated to promoting his research, to demonstrating that vegetarianism had a long and august history, its arguments on behalf of compassion formulated through the millennia. He wanted to show that we weren't alone, that our words weren't the first or the last on this vital subject, and that we all had something to contribute.

And now he was gone. Some of my emotion at his passing was guilt: that I hadn't been able to recognize someone with whom I'd been acquainted for so long—or, more pointedly, that I hadn't bothered to take the time to really *look* at the photo. Why had I given so little time and why was I so sure that I wouldn't know this person? My glance and snap decision seemed the very reverse of what we might hope from our friends when we're in need. My visit to the hospital, therefore, even though the diagnosis and prognosis were unknown to me, was an attempt to look at him again, to "tell" Rynn that I'd *seen* him. But *had I*, this second time? Was this body—simply a breath and a heartbeat—really *him*? Rynn had lived for language and communication, and both were now absent. I couldn't shake my sense that the body in the hospital bed belonged to a memory of Rynn: conscious, verbal, standing up, present. I hadn't seen him in the photo and now he saw nothing. He was unfamiliar, *unheimlich*, even to himself.

Then again, as the previous few days had illustrated, it was possible we were all unknown to ourselves. For more than a week, Rynn had been that most generic of nobodies: "John Doe." He'd failed to show up at an animal rights conference in Brazil and the organizers had tried to contact him at his home, to no avail. Rynn's death, which was covered by all the major New York newspapers, reflected a fear many of us have: that even though we're surrounded by people in the metropolis, we remain essentially anonymous; that we may fall and no one is there to pick us up or miss us until it's too late; that we die unknown and alone. Thankfully, in Rynn's case other runners saw him collapse. They called 911 and tried to administer CPR. It was too late. Rynn had gone into cardiac arrest and he'd been starved of oxygen for too long. The Rynn I'd seen was, in fact, brain-dead: his heart and lungs artificially kept pumping so the family could be gathered and a decision made to turn the machines off, which they were the following day.

On December 31, I was among thousands who visited Prospect Park to watch the fireworks ring out the old and ring in the new. Some revelers were even taking part in a midnight run. It's probable that not one among us knew that, days earlier, a man had fallen near where we stood, and that that man was Rynn. In my imagination, the timeframe has likewise collapsed: the explosions and cheers as another year is ushered in rising over a silent body lying in the snow; hope restored and a life snuffed out; a beginning and an end.

A further cause for discomfort was that I knew intimately the park where he fell. I had run around it hundreds of times. Yet in my crisscrossing and circling of its pathways—in races, on ordinary training outings, even in practicing hill starts on the slope leading up to Grand Army Plaza—I'd never come across Rynn. How was it possible that this space could have denied us the possibility of our meeting one another?

As we in the running community thought about what happened to Rynn, we reflected that any one of us could have been him. Some of us had slipped and fallen, had narrowly avoided being floored by a bicyclist or a car, or had found ourselves breathless and out of sorts miles from home. Like him, we'd left the house for a short run with no ID, with nary a thought that anything could go wrong so close to home.

But I saw myself in Rynn more intensely. Like me, he loved words—relished and savored them and hoped his audience would digest them with as much delight as he composed them. And both of us wanted people to read them and change. An independent scholar who preferred to use *anthropophagy* when *cannibalism* would suffice, Rynn was a human John Soane Museum—full of recesses, nooks, and alcoves where antiquities nestled, painstakingly labeled and precisely catalogued, to be dusted off and displayed for a public that might not appreciate them as much as the curator, but who were nonetheless irresistibly drawn to his house of curiosities. Both of us were a little out of our times, I fancy. We each enjoyed it when, in his susurrant wheeze, Rynn would offer to "inscribe" my "tome" rather than "sign" my "book." Why do the latter when the former was so much more fun to proffer?

We had resisted the allure of the academy (or perhaps weren't willing to undergo the hours or the discipline to become "genuine" scholars). We were too proud to submit to the rigors and humiliations of trying to get our writings published by large houses (or believed we wouldn't be properly appreciated or compensated by them). We were vegans and runners, and could be accused of asserting too much for either as vehicles for transformation. We were asthmatics and knew that desperate grasping for breath, the tension in the shoulders and across the chest that made every inhalation a labor and exhalation a gamble that the next intake of breath wouldn't fail. A few weeks before Rynn died I had ventured out with some faster runners and found myself forced to turn back because the frigid, dry air of a New York winter made it hard for me to breathe. Why hadn't Rynn done the same that snowy day?

An inhaler would never have been enough to compensate for the pressure on his heart.

Immediately following Rynn's death, a vegan running friend of mine anxiously emailed me and asked whether I knew of any pre-existing conditions that Rynn suffered from, since she was worried that non-vegans would blame his diet for his death, or at least question the notion that veganism was good for you.

My friend, who credited her diet and running with placing her cancer in remission, has all the self-belief and passionate intensity of someone who was given a terrible diagnosis and even worse prognosis, and survived. Not having been in such a situation, I can only imagine how miraculous it must seem to escape from that fate and how understandable it is to believe that a vegan diet and/or an intense fitness regimen, such as long-distance running, saved your life. And perhaps it did hers. But it would be dishonest to claim that either veganism or running, in combination or separately, is a panacea. Too many other factors are at play. All we can honestly say is that running and veganism may reduce the risks for certain ailments across a general population.

A case in point is Bud Burdick, a Brooklyn-based vegan athlete, who wrote on his blog (budburdick.com) on February 22, 2013:

> So I have this thing. It is not a nice thing, coming in and out of my life unwanted and undesired. It is an evil thing and it wishes to do me harm. Many battles have been fought and techniques tried, yet this thing continues to crawl its way back into my life. I have a whole army backing me up in many ways, yet this thing stays strong and continues to make its presence known.

I am not referring to something that is afflicting me from the outside world. This thing attacks me from the inside and wreaks havoc on my body and my system. This nuisance is a plague, a disease, an enemy. This thing is leukemia.

Bud had been diagnosed with the disease in July 2012. This was his last post. He died in April 2013. He was twenty-eight years old.

Ten days after Rynn passed, his half-brother Peter, younger than Rynn by eight years, collapsed from a heart attack while running in Central Park in Manhattan. He was sixty years old. Peter, according to his obituary in *The New York Times*, was like Rynn "a scholar, bibliophile and reader on all subjects," and "read Latin and ancient Greek for pleasure." He was also "a member of the Yale Varsity Squash Team, an A-ranked player in the New York Metropolitan Squash League, a lifelong advanced practitioner of yoga, and a tireless bicycle rider throughout the City." Their father, Rynn Berry, Sr., had died peacefully in his sleep in 2011 aged ninety-six; Rynn's mother had also lived into her nineties; and Peter's mother was still alive. What price the parsing of reasons why a man who ate no meat or dairy, and didn't smoke or drink, and his brother, who more than maintained his fitness, should die relatively prematurely, where their father lived almost to a hundred years?

Perhaps, in the end, it was just too cold.

IN THE WAKE of Rynn's death, I find myself struggling to forge the connections between veganism and running that came relatively easily to me as I conceptualized this book, and about which I write in the introduction. Or rather, I know the connections exist. It's simply that death, our constant companion, tends to overwhelm the organized consolations of philosophy or, for that matter, beliefs in one's own fitness and endurance.

Incomprehension at our lot and the recognition of our frailty are, of course, nothing new. The Book of Ecclesiastes is one long lamentation at the insubstantiality and inconsequence of human existence. The Psalmist and Jesus lament their forsakenness when confronted with their agonies. God gives Job no answer or justification for his suffering and Krishna refuses to release Arjuna from the terrible obligations of war.

Rynn, a scholar of Asian religious traditions, would have pointed out that material existence might be temporary but the soul continues its migrations through bodies until it no longer has to incarnate. He might have noted that the stopping of his heart should remind us that for sixty-eight years it had faithfully beaten the blood around his body and brain without complaint or only a passing awareness on his behalf—except perhaps for those moments when he ran and he could feel the heart pumping in time to the beat of his shoes on the asphalt. To weigh the long stretches of his life against, what one hopes, was an instantaneous loss of consciousness is to admit that, unlike Bud Burdick, Rynn had it lucky. He might have also observed that unlike the many other animals whose suffering he was deeply committed to alleviating or ending, his last moments had been in the open air, free to do what he loved and what his body craved.

One response to Bud, Peter, and Rynn's death is to proclaim "all things in moderation": a little bit of animal flesh or cream here, a little bit of running there; a life of simple pleasures, easily achievable and encompassable joys, and a withdrawal from anything that offers too large a claim on either ourselves or others, or the nature of the universe. Why literally and metaphorically go the extra mile? In pursuing these regimens to extremes, one might add, aren't vegans and/or runners in fact in quixotic flight *from* something: the reality of our deaths and the deaths of other animals, sometimes at the jaws or claws of species other than our own; the truth that our individual efforts to stave off the inevitable are fruitless, even fantastical? Eat, drink, and be stationary: for tomorrow we die.

Perhaps. Yet the soul and sole resist such constraints, not because we want to punish ourselves or demand more of others, but because we want to widen the ambit of what we can feel and do: to imagine an end-state that contains more possibilities than existed in our imaginations; to dream of a world where other creatures are no longer wholly constrained by our needs and desires. We know the odds are long, perhaps impossible. We know we might fall en route. But not to try. . . .

Rynn's books were dedicated to illustrating that vegetarianism was not new or a passing fad, but an ancient heritage worth honoring and preserving. In constructing his body of work, Rynn was passing on as well as passing through, another link in a chain reaching back to German philosopher Karl Jaspers' semi-mythic Axial Age of the Buddha, Mahavira, and Pythagoras, when human societies reoriented themselves toward systems of thought whose outlines can still be traced 2,500 years later.

That many of the ideas in favor of animal well-being and vegetarianism voiced then remain essentially the same today is both a ratification that they're valid and have stood the test of time and a recognition that, as Ecclesiastes 1:9 sighs, there really is nothing new under the sun. Humankind remains stubbornly resistant to a message that only gains more urgency as we move deeper and more decisively into the Anthropocene era. Whether the human race survives this particular time-trial may well depend on choices about food and our relationship to the world around us inscribed in Rynn's corpus and ours.

And so we keep going, this book a link with Rynn's legacy, as it is to *Cooking, Eating, Thinking*, as that is to Heidegger, and all the way back to the ancient Greeks: the bet that knowledge illuminates, our choices matter, and a hope (absurd, perhaps, but necessary to keep hold of) that, in the long run, the pathway will open up to reveal another turn ahead.

Acknowledgments

First of all, I must offer a big thank you to the contributors to this volume, many of whom I've had the pleasure of getting to know better through compiling this work, and some of whom I've been fortunate to run with both *à deux* and with members of their own running groups.

All anthologies—especially one as speculative and idiosyncratic as this one—leave out voices that might have been included. My hope is that this collection inspires others to think and write about, and perhaps take up, running and veganism. However, I'd be remiss if I didn't acknowledge some vegan runners not in this anthology who've inspired me. One is my good friend Amy Trakinski, who ran the New York City marathon four times and who'd most likely aver that neither running nor veganism is so complicated that philosophical maundering is required for either. Another is Joe Connelly, fellow vegan publisher, whose devotion to running contributed substantially to my own interest in the pastime. I wish to express my appreciation for the wisdom and support of Caryn Ginsberg, with whom I've had several years of pleasurable discussion about running. And finally, I'm delighted by the opportunity (admittedly in sad circumstances) to have gotten to know Cristina Abreu-Suzuki, whose dedication to the work and memory of Rynn

Berry is a testament to her fervor for veganism and her conviction that books matter.

I also want to thank the many enthusiastic members of the South Brooklyn Running Club, whom I've accompanied on many outings and who've helped me complete the yards when they were hardest. It's been a pleasure to get to know and spend time with them.

Running, Eating, Thinking benefited greatly from the careful and considered work of Wendy Lee, erstwhile editor at Lantern, and the invaluable skills of Kara Davis in production and Joe Lops in design. I'd like to thank Ruth Heidrich and Paul Shapiro for their kind words and support, and their own passionate commitment to the health of the planet, other animals, and themselves.

Finally, none of what I do on a daily basis—whether running or eating vegan food or writing—would be possible without the counsel, insight, and cajoling of my life partner, Mia MacDonald. She is the spring in my step.

Bibliography and Resources

Books by Contributors

Baur, Gene. *Farm Sanctuary: Changing Hearts and Minds About Animals and Food.* New York: Touchstone, 2008.

Frazier, Matt. *No Meat Athlete: Run on Plants and Discover Your Fittest, Fastest, Happiest Self.* Beverly, Mass.: Fair Winds Press, 2013.

Jaffe Jones, Ellen. *Eat Vegan on $4 a Day: A Game Plan for the Budget Conscious Cook.* Summertown, Tenn.: Book Publishing Company, 2011.

——. *Kitchen Divided: Vegan Dishes for Semi-Vegan Households.* Summertown, Tenn.: Book Publishing Company, 2013.

Jaffe Jones, Ellen and Alan Roettinger. *Paleo Vegan: Plant-Based Primal Recipes.* Summertown, Tenn.: Book Publishing Company, 2014.

McWilliams, James E. *A Revolution in Eating: How the Quest for Food Shaped America.* New York: Columbia University Press, 2005.

——. *Just Food: Where Locavores Get It Wrong and How We Can Truly Eat Responsibly.* Boston: Back Bay Books, 2009.

——. *The Politics of the Pasture: How Two Cattle Inspired a National Debate about Eating Animals.* New York: Lantern Books, 2013.

Patrick-Goudreau, Colleen. *On Being Vegan: Reflections on a Compassionate Life.* Montali Press, 2013.

———. *The 30-Day Vegan Challenge: The Ultimate Guide to Eating Cleaner, Getting Leaner, and Living Compassionately.* New York: Ballantine, 2011.

———. *Vegan's Daily Companion: 365 Days of Inspiration for Cooking, Eating, and Living Compassionately.* Beverly, Mass.: Fair Winds Press, 2011.

———. *The Vegan Table: 200 Unforgettable Recipes for Entertaining Every Guest at Every Occasion.* Beverly, Mass.: Fair Winds Press, 2009.

Rowe, Martin. *The Elephants in the Room: An Excavation.* New York: Lantern Books. 2013.

———. *The Polar Bear in the Zoo: A Speculation.* New York: Lantern Books, 2013.

Rowe, Martin and Ruth Heidrich. *Lifelong Running: Overcome the 11 Myths About Running and Life a Healthier Life.* New York: Lantern Books, 2013.

Running and Thinking

Austin, Michael W., ed. *Running & Philosophy: A Marathon for the Mind.* Oxford: Blackwell Publishing, 2007.

Brazier, Brendan. *Thrive: The Vegan Nutrition Guide to Optimal Performance in Sports and Life.* New York: Penguin, 2007.

———. *Thrive Fitness: The Vegan-Based Training Program for Maximum Strength, Health, and Fitness.* Cambridge, Mass.: Da Capo Press, 2009.

Dreyer, Danny and Katherine Dreyer. *ChiRunning: A Revolutionary*

Approach to Effortless, Injury-Free Running. New York: Touchstone, 2009.

Finn, Adharanand. *Running with the Kenyans: Discovering the Secrets of the Fastest People on Earth.* New York: Ballantine, 2012.

Galloway, Jeff. *Running: Getting Started.* London: Meyer & Meyer Sport, 2005.

Heidrich, Ruth E. *A Race for Life: The Amazing Story of How One Woman Survived Breast Cancer to Take on the Toughest Races in the World.* New York: Lantern Books, 2000.

——. *Senior Fitness: The Diet and Exercise Program for Maximum Health and Longevity.* New York, Lantern Books, 2005.

Heidrich, Ruth E. and Martin Rowe. *Lifelong Running: Overcome the 11 Myths About Running and Life a Healthier Life.* New York: Lantern Books, 2013. Jurek, Scott and Steve Friedman. *Eat and Run: My Unlikely Journey to Ultramarathon Greatness.* Boston: Houghton Mifflin Harcourt, 2012.

McDougall, Christopher. *Born to Run: A Hidden Tribe, Superathletes, and the Greatest Race the World Has Never Seen.* New York: Knopf, 2009.

Mipham, Sakyong. *Running with the Mind of Meditation: Lessons for Training Body and Mind.* New York: Three Rivers Press, 2012.

Murakami, Haruki. *What I Talk About When I Talk About Running.* New York: Random House, 2007.

Pfitzinger, Pete and Scott Douglas. *Advanced Marathoning.* Champaign, Ill.: Human Kinetics, 2001.

Robbins, Liz. *A Race Like No Other: 26.2 Miles Through the Streets of New York.* New York: HarperCollins, 2008.

Roll, Rich. *Finding Ultra: Rejecting Middle Age, Becoming One of the World's Fittest Men, and Discovering Myself.* New York: Crown, 2012.

Sheehan, George. *The Essential Sheehan: A Lifetime of Running Wisdom from the Legendary Dr. George Sheehan.* New York: Rodale, 2013.

———. *Running & Being: The Total Experience.* New York: Rodale, 1978 [2013].

Eating and Thinking

Adams, Carol J. *The Sexual Politics of Meat: A Feminist-Vegetarian Critical Theory*, 20th Anniversary Edition. New York: Continuum, 2010.

Allhoff, Fritz and Dave Monroe. *Food & Philosophy: Eat, Think and Be Merry.* Oxford: Blackwell Publishing, 2007.

Berry, Rynn. *Famous Vegetarians and Their Favorite Recipes.* New York: Pythagorean Publications, 1993.

———. *Food for the Gods: Vegetarianism and the World's Religions.* New York: Pythagorean Publications, 1998.

———. *Hitler: Neither Vegetarian Nor Animal Lover.* New York: Pythagorean Publications, 2004.

Burkett, Denis. *Don't Forget Fibre in Your Diet.* London: Collins, 1979.

Curtin, Deane W. and Lisa M. Heldke, eds. *Cooking, Eating, Thinking: Transformative Philosophies of Food.* Bloomington: Indiana University Press, 1992.

Davis, Brenda, Vesanto Melina, and Rynn Berry. *Becoming Raw: The Essential Guide to Raw Vegan Diets.* Summertown, Tenn.: Book Publishing Company, 2010

Kaplan, David M. *The Philosophy of Food.* Berkeley: University of California Press, 2012.

Pollan, Michael. *In Defense of Food: An Eater's Manifesto*. New York: Penguin, 2008.

———. *The Omnivore's Dilemma: A Natural History of Four Meals*. New York: Penguin, 2007.

Sattilaro, Anthony J. *Recalled by Life*. New York: Avon, 1984.

Stone, Gene, ed. *Forks Over Knives: The Plant-Based Way to Health*. New York: The Experiment, 2011.

Resources (all links were active as of February 3, 2014)

Active.com: <http://www.active.com>. A website that lists races in your community as well as everywhere else.

Brighter Green: <www.brightergreen.org>. A public policy "action" tank exploring the effect of intensive animal agriculture around the world on climate change, public health, animal welfare, resource depletion and conservation, and equity.

Facebook: Vegan Runners Group: <https://www.facebook.com/groups/438769342893624/>

Fat, Sick, and Nearly Dead: <http://www.fatsickandnearlydead.com>.

Forks Over Knives: <http://www.forksoverknives.com>

Great Vegan Athletes: http://www.greatveganathletes.com/

James Porteous, Vegan Running Coach: <http://plantendurancecoaching.com/>

Marathon Guide: <http://www.marathonguide.com/>. A site that lists all the marathons around the world by month, with comments from runners on each race.

National Black Marathoners Association: <http://www.blackmarathoners.org/>. Self-explanatory.

No Meat Athlete: <http://www.nomeatathlete.com/>

Runner's World <www.runnersworld.org>

Running Vegan: <http://www.runningvegan.com/>

Ruth Heidrich: <http://www.ruthheidrich.com/>. Ruth Heidrich's website.

Vegan Fitness: <http://www.veganfitness.net/home/>

Vegan Runners UK: <http://www.veganrunners.org.uk/>

Vegucated: <http://www.getvegucated.com>

Veggie Runners: <http://www.veggierunners.com/>

About the Contributors

GENE BAUR is the co-founder and president of Farm Sanctuary, America's leading farm animal protection organization. He is the bestselling author of *Farm Sanctuary: Changing Hearts and Minds about Animals and Food* (Touchstone, 2008).

CATHERINE BERLOT is an M.D. and Ph.D. with a specialization in cellular and molecular biology.

CASSANDRA GREENWALD is a writer and editor. She studied creative writing and graduated from the Evergreen State College and later went on to learn about the theory and art of cooking in culinary school and restaurants. She frequently combines her focus on the written word and her passion for the kitchen to test and edit cookbook recipes. She lives in Chicago with her partner and their cat named Bear. Her website is editcassandra.com.

JL FIELDS is a vegan cook, lifestyle coach, and educator—certified by the Main Street Vegan Academy. She is co-author of *Vegan for Her: The Woman's Guide to Being Healthy and Fit on a Plant-Based Diet* (Da Capo Press, 2013) with Virginia Messina. A devoted culinary student, JL has studied at the Natural Gourmet Institute and

Organic Avenue, and completed the Intensive Study Program at The Christina Pirello School of Natural Cooking and Integrative Health Studies. Her website is jlgoesvegan.com.

MATT FRAZIER is a vegan runner who recently completed his first 100-mile ultramarathon. He is the author of *No Meat Athlete: Run on Plants and Discover Your Fittest, Fastest, Happiest Self* (Fair Winds Press, 2013), based on his hugely popular blog NoMeat-Athlete.com, which attracts 170,000 unique visitors a month. His newsletter has more than 30,000 subscribers, and his Facebook page has received more than 50,000 "Likes." Matt is regularly featured regularly in running magazines, websites, and books, including *Thrive Foods* by Brendan Brazier and *Finding Ultra* by Rich Roll. He lives in Asheville, North Carolina. His website is NoMeatAthlete.com.

CHRISTINE FRIETCHEN is a digital content consultant at Random House. She loves to sew, run, swim, and write. Originally from Leavenworth, Kansas, she currently lives in Brooklyn, New York.

GORDON E. HARVEY is a professor of history and head of the history and foreign languages department at Jacksonville State University, Alabama—his home state. A specialist in the recent U.S. South and its politics, Dr. Harvey has published several articles, historical journals, and essays in edited works, including an essay on the politics of environmental protection in modern Florida in *Paradise Lost? The Environmental History of Florida*, edited by Ray

Arsenault and Jack Davis (University Press of Florida, 2005). His website is thisrunninglife.wordpress.com.

ELLEN JAFFE JONES is a certified personal trainer (AFAA), running coach (RRCA), and accomplished endurance and sprint runner. She is the author of the bestseller *Eat Vegan on $4 a Day* and *The Kitchen Divided: Vegan Dishes for Semi-Vegan Households*. She spent eighteen years in television news as a consumer/investigative reporter and morning anchor. She has won two Emmys, including one for a story that led to an FDA food recall, and the National Press Club Award for Consumer Reporting. She spent five years at Smith Barney where she was the number-one market performer in her branch in 2001, and in the top 10 in 2002; the only woman on the list both years. The website Great Vegan Athletes has honored her among the top vegan female runners. When not on book tour, Ellen loves to volunteer coach high school girls' cross-country and track. Her website is vegcoach.com.

JAMES MCWILLIAMS is a historian and writer based in Austin, Texas. His books include *Just Food: Where Locavores Get It Wrong and How We Can Truly Eat Responsibly*, *A Revolution in Eating: How the Quest for Food Shaped America*, and *The Politics of the Pasture: How Two Cattle Inspired a National Debate about Eating Animals*. His writing on food, agriculture, and animals has appeared in the *New York Times*, *Harper's*, *The Washington Post*, *Slate*, *Forbes*, *Travel and Leisure*, *The Los Angeles Times*, *The International Herald Tribune*, *The Christian Science Monitor*, and *The Texas Observer*, where he is a contributing writer. He blogs at james-mcwilliams.com.

LISETTE OROPESA has appeared in more than 100 performances at the Metropolitan Opera and has sung many major roles there, including Susanna in Mozart's *The Marriage of Figaro* and Gilda in Verdi's *Rigoletto*, as well as having appeared in eight of the Met's Live! in HD productions. She has sung various leading roles in both the U.S. and Europe: at the Bayerische Staatsoper, the Welsh National Opera, ABAO Opera Bilbao, the San Francisco Opera, the Santa Fe Opera, and the Ravinia Festival, to name a few. Along with her blossoming operatic career, her fitness journey has been featured in several publications, including *Runner's World* magazine and *Classical Singer* magazine. Her website is lisetteoropesa.com.

Addressing the spiritual, social, and practical aspects of a compassionate lifestyle, COLLEEN PATRICK-GOUDREAU is the author of five books, including the award-winning *The Joy of Vegan Baking*, *The Vegan Table*, *Color Me Vegan*, and *Vegan's Daily Companion*. She is also the creator of the life-changing online multimedia program *The 30-Day Vegan Challenge* (30dayveganchallenge.com) and the host and producer of the popular podcast, *Vegetarian Food for Thought*. She has appeared on the Food Network and PBS and is a contributor to National Public Radio and *The Christian Science Monitor*. Her website is compassionatecook.com.

KIMATNI D. RAWLINS is the Founder of Fit Fathers, an inspirational movement encouraging dads to mobilize family values toward healthier eating and daily exercise through various activities. Kimatni's motto is simple: "Health, fitness and nutrition are priorities for the extension of life. Stay active, eat well and constantly energize yourself." His website is FitFathers.com.

MARTIN ROWE is the publisher at Lantern Books. He is the author of *The Polar Bear in the Zoo: A Speculation* and *The Elephants in the Room: An Excavation*, and co-author with Ruth Heidrich of *Lifelong Running: Overcome the 11 Myths About Running and Life a Healthier Life* (all Lantern Books, 2013). He is also the editor of *The Way of Compassion: Vegetarianism, Environmentalism, Animal Advocacy, and Social Justice* (Stealth Technologies, 1999) and *Nicaea: A Book of Correspondences* (Lindisfarne, 2003). As of April 2014, he has run sixteen marathons and thirty-three half-marathons. He lives in Brooklyn, New York. His website is martin-rowe.com.

JASMIN SINGER is the co-founder and Executive Director of Our Hen House (www.ourhenhouse.org), a multimedia hub of opportunities to change the world for animals. Jasmin is also the co-host, along with her partner Mariann Sullivan, of the award-winning Our Hen House podcast, as well as the Our Hen House TV show, which is part of Brooklyn Independent Media. With Our Hen House, Jasmin produces an online magazine and an eBook publishing arm called Hen Press. She has appeared on *The Dr. Oz Show, HuffPo Live*, as well as in the documentaries *The Ghosts in Our Machine* and *Vegucated*, and in a national commercial for *Fat, Sick, and Nearly Dead*. She is the former campaigns manager for Farm Sanctuary, and has presented widely on the subjects of animal rights and veganism. Jasmin and Mariann live in New York City with their pit bull, Rose.

SCOTT SPITZ is a drug-free, anarchist, metal-head, twenty-year vegan and father. He has a half-marathon personal record of 1:09:46 and a marathon PR of 2:25:55. He started running when he was about six years old. His website is runvegan.wordpress.com. Scott is currently undergoing treatment for stomach cancer.

About the Publisher

LANTERN BOOKS was founded in 1999 on the principle of living with a greater depth and commitment to the preservation of the natural world. In addition to publishing books on animal advocacy, vegetarianism, religion, and environmentalism, Lantern is dedicated to printing books in the U.S. on recycled paper and saving resources in day-to-day operations. Lantern is honored to be a recipient of the highest standard in environmentally responsible publishing from the Green Press Initiative.

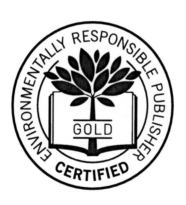

www.lanternbooks.org

CPSIA information can be obtained
at www.ICGtesting.com
Printed in the USA
FFOW05n2108150514

9 781590 563489